Private Eye, Heart and Hip

WITHDRAWN FROM
THE LIBRARY

UNIVERSITY OF
WINCHESTER

D1145813

For Churchill Livingstone:
Publisher: Peter Richardson
Copy Editor: Penelope Lyons
Production Controller: Nora Cameron
Design Direction: Sarah Cape
Marketing Executive: Louise Ashworth

Private Eye, Heart & Hip

Surgical consultants, the National
Health Service and private medicine

John Yates PhD MHSM DipHSM
Honorary Research Fellow, University of Birmingham,
Birmingham, UK

CHURCHILL LIVINGSTONE
EDINBURGH HONG KONG LONDON MADRID MELBOURNE NEW YORK AND
TOKYO 1995

CHURCHILL LIVINGSTONE
Medical Division of Pearson Professional Limited

Distributed in the United States of America by Churchill Livingstone Inc.,
650 Avenue of the Americas, New York, N.Y. 10011, and by associated
companies, branches and representatives throughout the world.

© Pearson Professional Limited 1995

All rights reserved. No part of this publication may be reproduced, stored in a
retrieval system, or transmitted in any form or by any means, electronic,
mechanical, photocopying recording or otherwise, without either the prior
permission of the publishers (Churchill Livingstone, Robert Stevenson
House, 1-3 Baxter's Place, Leith Walk, Edinburgh, EH1 3AF), or a licence
permitting restricted copying in the United Kingdom issued by the Copyright
Licensing Agency Ltd, 90 Tottenham Court Road, London, W19 9HE.

First published 1995

ISBN 0–443–05466–5

British Library Cataloguing in Publication Data
A catalogue record for this book is available from the British Library

Library of Congress Cataloging in Publication Data
A catalog record for this book is available from the Library of Congress

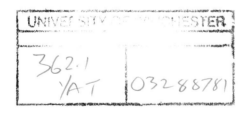
UNIVERSITY OF MANCHESTER

362.1
/AT   03288781

The right of John Yates to be identified as author of this Work has been asserted
by him in accordance with the Copyright, Designs and Patents Act 1988.

The
publisher's
policy is to use
paper manufactured
from sustainable forests

Printed by Bell and Bain Ltd, Glasgow

Contents

Preface

When I discussed this book with my publishers, they asked who was the intended audience for the book and what would be the benefit to the audience. The first question was easy to answer; the book is aimed at surgeons, managers and politicians, but the second question posed a problem. If I am honest, those who seriously take up the challenges will encounter considerable hardship and the ultimate beneficiaries will not be the professionals but the patients.

The preliminary results of this research work were portrayed in a Channel 4 documentary and the response to the programme was almost overwhelming. For weeks I received letters from staff giving examples of the inequity of the Health Service, but the most staggering response came from the patients. There were letters that simply said 'thank you for raising the issue' and many heart rending examples of the pain, frustration and bitterness felt by many people who could not afford to pay for jumping NHS waiting lists. The support and gratitude received was quite touching, one patient even sent a cake!

Birmingham 1995   J.M.Y.

Acknowledgements

I have received help and support from many doctors, managers and academics, but particularly from half a dozen surgical friends, who have constructively criticised sections of my work. My so called 'attack' on the medical profession is strongly supported by a significant section of that profession. One consultant surgeon wrote to me saying "This whole subject is dear to my heart, indeed I tried to write something along similar lines a couple of years ago but could not get it published as I wished to use a pseudonym". Another doctor said to me "I have wanted to say this since I was a houseman."

This research work was sponsored by The Joseph Rowntree Charitable Trust, who reacted quickly and generously when I outlined the contrast in waiting times experienced by the wealthy and less wealthy in our society. It could not have been completed without the close support of my immediate colleagues, who have taken on extra work within the unit in order that I could spend 'substantially the whole of my time' on this subject. My thanks go to Mike Davidge, Sue Elias, Mike Harley, Bob Jayes, Lorna Vickerstaff and Kate Wood for keeping the unit afloat whilst my attention was on this subject.

Finally, I need to thank Chris, David, Ron, Keith and friends - the suburban guerrillas.

To all those who have helped I am very grateful. We have clearly touched a raw nerve in the NHS.

Investigating the situation

CONTENTS

1

Divided cities

Some cities have clear divisions which segregate groups of their citizens. Beirut has a green line, Berlin was divided by a wall and Belfast still is. My adopted city has been spared obvious physical segregation, but it has a deep division. When I came to live in the city, over 20 years ago, I was unaware of it, but as time has passed the division has become more and more apparent. The health care offered to its citizens has become less determined by need, and increasingly determined by the patient's ability to pay. Birmingham is divided by money.

In the richer suburbs, a visit to the general practitioner can result in a stark choice. If my general practitioner decided I needed to see an ophthalmologist he would ask me, 'Are you insured?' He has two lists of telephone numbers and addresses. The first list is for those who have private insurance or can afford to pay for their treatment. Those patients will wait only a week or two to see a consultant in a quiet, well-upholstered consulting room. If an operation is needed it will follow in a couple of weeks and will always be undertaken by a highly trained consultant surgeon. As I do not have private insurance, the general practitioner will choose from a second list of National Health Service (NHS) hospitals. He will send a referral letter to one of the hospitals that has an ophthalmology out-patient clinic. I need not be surprised if I have to wait 30–50 weeks for an appointment, just to see the surgeon. The clinics will be huge and the time spent with each patient will be limited. For those needing an operation, a further wait of about a year may be expected and over half of the operations will be performed by a trainee surgeon.

WHAT'S NEW?

Waiting a long time for an out-patient appointment and, subsequently, an operation are not new experiences for those who live in Birmingham. In the early 1970s, out-patient waiting times were enormous and in-patient waiting lists were numbered in thousands. The city had only 6 consultant ophthalmologists whilst Glasgow, a city of similar size, had 13. I was part of a team opening a new ward block in one of the city's district general hospitals. It had a new purpose-built ophthalmology ward and operating theatre. We found it difficult to get advice about how to equip and open the new unit.

The ophthalmologists of the city were not supportive of the establishment of a separate unit in a district general hospital and wanted to maintain and expand a single-site specialist hospital for the city. The lack of support showed itself in the reticence to provide professional advice for preparing job descriptions and advertisements for a new consultant post. There was even an unwillingness to provide an assessor for the interview and we suspected the job was virtually 'blacked' by the profession. The eventual appointee was not welcomed into the 'fold' and the unit remained isolated, underdeveloped and underused for years. At the time, I could not understand why the ophthalmologists were so reluctant to participate in what I thought would offer some improvement in the services we could offer to our patients.

A decade later, a British Medical Association survey revealed that in September 1984 the average wait for a routine ophthalmology appointment in England was 15 weeks (Yates & Wood

1985). In the West Midlands the average figure was 22 weeks, but in Birmingham's main ophthalmology unit the minimum wait was over 34 weeks. Two years later, some hospitals had resorted to underlining in red the year on the appointment card to stop patients from coming a year early. Others simply did not send out appointment cards because the date would be 2–4 years hence. Newspaper stories in the city included evidence that one person had lost his sight whilst waiting for an out-patient appointment. At one time in 1986 the main eye hospital had 2362 general practitioners' letters stacked in the medical records office requesting appointments for patients, and the estimated wait for an appointment was between 37 and 60 weeks. In 1988, a manager's report at the same hospital stated that the waiting time had reached 65 weeks and was worsening. For one consultant the wait was over 100 weeks. For the last 12 years it has been difficult to get an appointment in less than 6 months, and almost impossible to be seen in under 3 months except in cases of extreme urgency. The only occasions on which routine appointments were available in less than 3 months were when a newly appointed surgeon had taken up post and his new clinics had just commenced (Fig. 1.1).

Throughout the early 1980s the waiting list at the main hospital for in-patient admission always exceeded 1000 patients and at any time the list would have half of its patients waiting over a year for admission. The 1980s saw the introduction of the National Waiting List Initiative and substantial managerial and political effort, together with additional resources, was put into reducing in-patient waiting lists and waiting time. At the beginning of the initiative in 1986, consideration was even given to sending Birmingham patients to London for treatment in order to reduce waiting time (Anon. 1986). Today, the Patients' Charter standard insists the NHS ensures that no patient waits more than 18 months on the in-patient waiting list for a cataract operation. Undoubtedly, 8 years of initiatives have led to improvements in in-patient waiting time, but this improved situation can still be preceded by a wait of 30–50 weeks just to see an ophthalmologist at an out-patient clinic.

These waiting problems rarely excite the interest of the media. Even if facts are presented which show that the problem is one faced by thousands of elderly residents of the city, there are numerous reasons and excuses offered to minimize the impact of

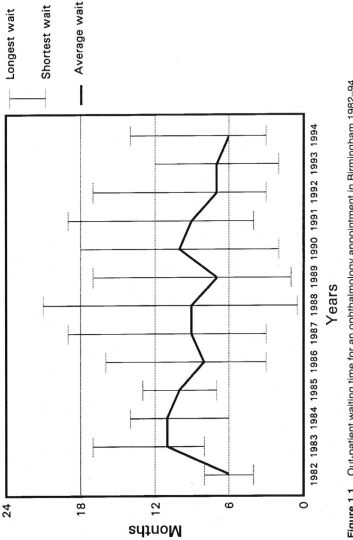

Figure 1.1 Out-patient waiting time for an ophthalmology appointment in Birmingham 1982–94

Source:
Health Authority Information Sheets sent to general practitioners

the story. The surgeons and managers are faced by shortages of resources, poor conditions, bottlenecks of inefficiency and an apparently never-ending demand from a growing number of elderly. Health officials are quick to point out how speedily the urgent cases are dealt with, how well so many thousands of others (the more urgent) are treated and how few patients complain. Future plans are often cited to explain how performance will improve and then reduce waiting time. Today's difficulties will be overcome when tomorrow arrives.

Long waiting times seem to remain part of Birmingham's normal experience. The only way to change the situation is to reach for your wallet. Twenty years ago, only a very small proportion of patients were insured or paid to be treated privately. In effect, it was only the very rich who jumped the queue. Today, the proportions are quite different. Despite more surgeons and an increased investment in expensive equipment by the NHS, the average citizen has seen little improvement in waiting time. The increasing number of people who do wait a shorter period of time, do so only because they are able and prepared to pay for treatment. In contrast to those patients who in Figure 1.1 had to wait for 3–12 months, those who could afford to pay were seen in 1 or 2 weeks. In the early 1970s, with only half a dozen ophthalmologists and few people paying for private insurance, the number of people who could avail themselves of a private appointment in 1 or 2 weeks would be quite small in number. Today, with 10 ophthalmologists, most of whom devote 2 half-days per week to seeing private patients in their consulting rooms, and surgeons from surrounding areas coming into Birmingham to help in the trade, we now have a large well-established business. It is, however, a service that simply is not available to a large proportion of the city's patients.

NOT JUST ONE SPECIALTY, NOR JUST ONE CITY

The problem is not one faced only by patients needing eye surgery in Birmingham – it is one experienced in other specialties and in other towns and cities. In Birmingham, waiting times in other specialties are not always as long as those found in ophthalmology, but waits of over 3 months are routinely experienced in dermatology, neurology, rheumatology, vascular clinics, ENT, neurosurgery and urology. In one specialty the problems are even greater than in ophthalmology. Birmingham's general practitioners have around 20 local orthopaedic surgeons to whom they can refer patients, but in nearly all NHS clinics long waiting times can be expected. In the autumn of 1994 I rang all the hospitals in Birmingham that had an orthopaedic out-patient clinic and asked for the latest waiting times. The range was from 4–115 weeks with an average wait of 33 weeks. Of 18 surgeons contacted only 4 could be seen within 3 months, but for 7 of them the wait was between 6 months and 2 years (Table 1.1). I rang the same surgeons' rooms seeking a private appointment; 2 did not see private patients but for the remaining 16, I was offered an appointment within 1–7 weeks. The average wait for a private appointment was just 3½ weeks.

The position in Birmingham is not untypical of the British NHS. The out-patient waiting times in many surgical specialties have been a hidden sore of the British NHS for years. From time to time, local and national newspapers give examples of unac-ceptably long waiting times. 73-year-old Megan Thompson of

Table 1.1 Waiting time for an orthopaedic appointment in Birmingham 1994

Surgeon	In an NHS Clinic	In private rooms
A	4	4
B	9	4
C	12	2
D	12	3
E	14	3
F	14	4
G	14	4
H	14	7
I	18	No PPs
J	21	3
K	23	1
L	28	6
M	30	2
N	48	4
O	52	4
P	70	6
Q	100	1
R	115	No PPs
Range	4–115	1–7
Average	33	3.5

Source:
Telephone enquiries to NHS hospitals and private rooms in Autumn 1994 (the information for NHS hospitals was sometimes out of date but it was the latest available to an enquiry made by a member of the public)

Cambridge was offered a 4-year wait to see an orthopaedic surgeon (Doyle 1994). Recognizing that even after that wait for an appointment she might still have to wait a further period before reaching the operating theatre she astutely observed, 'I could have been dead by the time of the operation.' Data about the first half of the patient's wait has not, until recently, been systematically recorded in this country. Surveys in 1984 and 1994 show a depressing picture.

Table 1.2 shows, in some specialties, that we wait much longer today than we did 10 years ago. These 'average' figures mask three important points.

1. These waiting times are for 'routine' appointments and urgent referrals are nearly always seen very much more quickly.
2. The averages always cover huge variations between clinics up and down the country. Figure 1.2 illustrates that some clinics can be found where there are waits of a month or less, but others where the wait is over a year. There is no pattern to these variations and long or short waiting times can occur anywhere in the country.
3. It is probably true to say that most people wait for less than the average times shown. In part, this is explained by the fact that many people drop out of queues because they get better, die or go privately.

No matter what the arguments are about the accuracy of the figures, there is no doubt that thousands of British citizens routinely wait months just to meet a consultant surgeon. There is

Table 1.2   Average waiting time for a routine NHS out-patient appointment in weeks 1984 and 1994

Specialty	1984	1994
Orthopaedics	16. 1	25. 4
Ophthalmology	15. 1	19. 3
General surgery	7. 9	13. 2
ENT	13. 6	14. 4

Source:
1984 Survey of minimum waiting time for routine appointments in 163 English districts (Yates & Wood 1985)
1994 Data from 4974 out-patient clinics in England and Wales given to the College of Health Help Line (Latest information available was at October 1994)
See text for discussion on interpretation of data

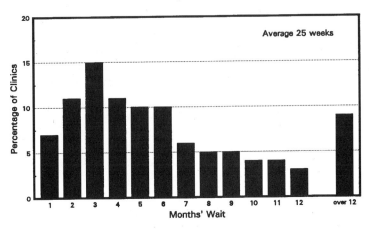

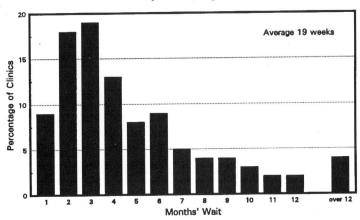

Figure 1.2 Out-patient waiting time in the NHS in England and Wales – orthopaedics and ophthalmology 1994

Source:
College of Health Helpline November 1994

an uncertainty during this period that worries many patients and GPs. The GP has sent the patient for a second and specialist opinion, and the patient has not been given a complete assurance about his illness. Quite often the worry is compounded by the fact that the patient is not even given a date for an appointment, but merely told that the wait could be many months; or perhaps there is no information at all about a date. In contrast to the way the NHS works, the private sector is much more speedy and precise.

To see if Birmingham was unusual, I surveyed 169 orthopaedic surgeons throughout the whole of England, and a further 66 ophthalmologists from London and selected provincial cities. The vast majority of surgeons could see private patients within 3 weeks. On only three occasions was there a wait of over 6 weeks and these were explained by the fact that the consultant was on holiday or other leave. Figure 1.3 shows the distribution of waiting times in the two specialties and can be compared with the waiting times in the NHS shown in Figure 1.2. When doing so, remember that the NHS data is measured in months and the private sector data is shown in weeks. To compare the two on the same scale you need to examine Figure 1.4. That diagram begins to show the inequality of access that upsets the man in the street. It uncovers the hidden part of Britain's two-tier waiting list – the wait just to see the surgeon. In specialties like orthopaedics, one sector offers 96% of patients an appointment within a month, but in the other sector less than 7% of patients get such an offer. The wait averages 2 weeks in the private sector or 25 weeks in the NHS – and only then can the patient join one of the most famous queues in the Western world – the British waiting list.

The waiting list is the most notorious feature of the British NHS – an apparently endless queue of patients awaiting an operation. When the NHS came into existence in 1948 there were half a million patients in the queue, but today that figure is over one million. In contrast to the steady increase in the total numbers waiting, an increase that has continued for the entire life of the NHS, recent years have seen a substantial decrease in the number of patients waiting over a year for admission. We are confused by the mixed messages that we receive. Whilst managers, academics and politicians can assure us that the length of the queue is unimportant, no matter how much they

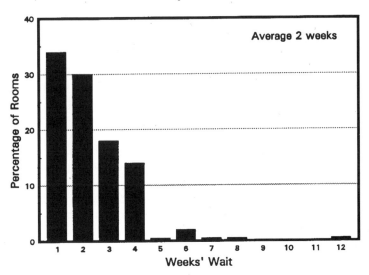

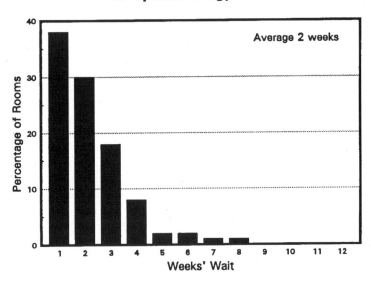

Figure 1.3 Out-patient waiting time in the private sector in England – orthopaedics and ophthalmology 1994

Source:
IACC Survey September 1994

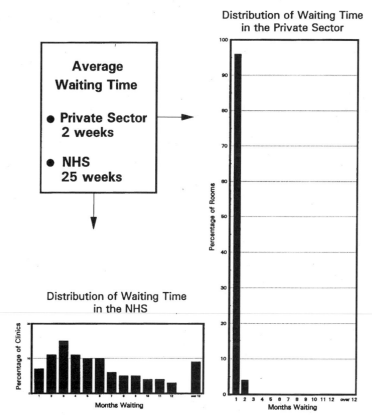

Figure 1.4 Contrasts in waiting time for an orthopaedics appointment – the NHS and the private sector 1994

Source:
Figures 1.2, 1.3

point to the reduction in the numbers waiting over a year for admission, at street level the vibes are different. The size of the waiting list is increasing all the time and anyone who has encountered a queue at the supermarket or on the motorway has a gut feeling that the longer the queue, the longer the wait.

The public also know that the in-patient waiting list only shows half the picture and that the NHS has consistently failed to gather information about out-patient waiting time – the hidden waiting list described earlier. The combined suspicion about the way politicians argue over waiting times and waiting numbers, and the fact that all concerned seem to ignore out-patient waiting time, leaves most people very sceptical. The reality remains that those who can afford private medicine continue to do so in order to jump one or both of the queues and thereby shorten their waiting time. Patient surveys (Higgins 1988, Primarolo 1994) confirm that acquiring a more speedy admission is the main reason for opting for private care and the major plank of the private sector's advertising strength is the statement, 'And we didn't have to wait'. The private sector openly admits that 'Waiting for elective surgery under the NHS is at the heart of decisions to purchase private medical insurance' (*Laing's Review of Private Healthcare* 1993).

It is a well known and fatalistically accepted characteristic of the NHS that those who can afford to pay are treated more quickly than those who cannot. What is less widely appreciated is that payment not only ensures faster treatment, but also more treatment. In recent years about 10% of the population have been insured for private medical care, but the proportion of planned operations (i.e. not emergency operations) carried out in the private sector is almost twice as great. In 1981, whilst only 7% of the population had private insurance (*Laing's Review of Private Healthcare* 1993), 13% of all planned operations were done privately (Nicholl et al 1984), and for some operations, such as hip replacements, 26% were carried out on private patients.

Some 5 years later (Nicholl et al 1989) the proportions were 9%, 17% and 28%. By 1991–92, 11% of the population were insured and the private sector claimed to be doing 20% of planned surgery (Anon. 1994a) and 30% of hip replacements (The British United Provident Association Ltd. 1994). The imbalance shown in Figure 1.5 is explained partly by the fact that some British citizens pay cash rather than use insurance cover (although not many), partly by the fact that foreign nationals come here for treatment, but mainly by the fact that those who can afford to pay get treated at a disproportionately higher rate than those who cannot afford to pay.

PHILOSOPHICAL AND POLITICAL DREAMS?

As the British emerged from the Second World War their politicians promised them that, 'Disease must be attacked in the poorest or in the richest, in the same way as the fire brigade will give full assistance to the humble cottage as readily as to the most

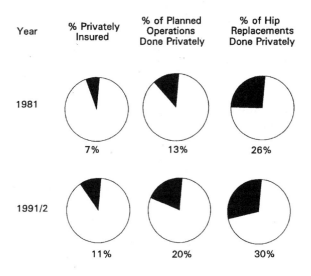

Year	% Privately Insured	% of Planned Operations Done Privately	% of Hip Replacements Done Privately
1981	7%	13%	26%
1991/2	11%	20%	30%

Figure 1.5 Comparing NHS and private care

important mansion' (Churchill, quoted 1976). Fifty years later, how does reality match the vision expressed by Winston Churchill?

Every single day there are British citizens worrying about how to cope with waiting for an out-patient appointment or an operation. Millions have now decided to take the worry out of waiting by insuring for private medical care, in an attempt to eliminate or minimize waiting times. Some resent having to pay twice for health care, but clearly feel the financial loss incurred is worthwhile. Each day, others who have not opted for private health insurance wrestle with their conscience or their bank balance to see if they too can find a way of spending £50 or £60 to get a rooms appointment, or save the thousands of pounds needed for some major operation. It is all a long way from the British health care system that was designed to provide equal access for all the people of Britain.

The philosophical and political ideals in British culture run counter to the reality faced by its citizens. The philosophy of the medical profession claims that it should be allowed to treat patients according to strict clinical criteria, unfettered by other considerations. Politicians of all political affiliations seek a class-less society, and across the political spectrum one can find considerable support for the early dreams of the British NHS. Despite all this support, there is evidence that the rich–poor divide is as great as it was in 1948. In *The Economist* it was suggested that, 'Not only is the income gap between rich and poor widening, so is the health gap. The National Health Service was supposed to make this unlikely, if not impossible. What has gone wrong? And what can be done about it?' (Anon. 1994b).

This was perhaps a little harsh on the NHS in expecting it to solve the health care problems of the nation on its own. An individual's health is influenced by four factors – genetic make-up, the environment in which that person lives, behaviour, and the health services that are available. The first three factors are dominant and are little influenced by the health service that is available. At birth, some of us have physical or mental defects that will be with us for the whole of our lives. Some of these, such as severe mental handicap or a major limb deformity are obvious at birth, but others reveal themselves at later stages. Our health is influenced by the environment into which we are born and where we live. Do we have a caring family? Do we suffer physical or mental abuse? Is the environment polluted by local industry? Do we live in insanitary conditions? Health is also influenced by how we behave. Even those with apparently identical genetic make-up who live in the same environment are likely to have poorer patterns of health and shorter lives if they smoke regularly, take drugs and alcohol and drive motorbikes without helmets.

The fourth component that influences our health is the health service that is available to us. To some extent it tries to influence the three main determinants by its effort to do research into things that will alter genetic make-up and by informing and leading campaigns on how to improve our environment and behaviour. Most of the role of the NHS, however, is clearing up the mess after genetic, environmental and behavioural factors have had their way. A health service in reality becomes an illness service, one that tries to cure diseases that become apparent. If it fails to cure, it tries to minimize the effects of disease and if it can do neither it finally tries to care for people, either until such time as a cure is available, or simply to provide comfort until death. A health service cannot, therefore, be solely blamed for inequalities in the health of the people it tries to serve. There is ample evidence to suggest that many of the variations in mortality and morbidity suffered by different groups within a population are caused by a combination of environmental and behavioural factors. But is there some link between the rich–poor divide, the inequality of waiting times and the structure of the health services provided in Britain?

COINCIDENCES?

Those who find themselves waiting for treatment, whilst others jump the queue, feel hurt. There is even anger about a system which is so inequitable and the anger leads to a search for scape-goats. Who can be blamed? How can surgeons, managers and politicians allow this inequality to occur? The British health care system has a state and a private sector that work side by side, using the same surgeons. Those surgeons who choose to work in both sectors can more than double their NHS salary. Are they greedy, incompetent or corrupt? Are the occasional allegations of fraud (for example, Chadda 1994a), mischievous and unfounded or the tip of an iceberg? If there were more surgeons with more resources, wouldn't the problem just disappear?

It is not clear who is responsible and the more paranoid among us might feel that there is a conspiracy between surgeons, managers and politicians that leaves patients suffering in silence. Nobody appears to be able to act as an advocate for patients and identify which, if any, of the three parties share any responsibility for this inequity. No-one has ever produced concrete evidence that gives any hint as to who is responsible for the failure of the system. Everybody knows that the rich jump the queue, but neither managers, surgeons nor politicians are held accountable for failing the poor. No-one produces convinc-ing evidence to answer these questions one way or the other. The patient is struck by five coincidences that don't seem to give the professionals any concern:

- the poor are more prone to illness and early death, and it is the poor who have to wait longest for treatment
- the regions that have the most private beds are those that have the worst waiting lists
- the specialties that have the longest waiting times are the ones that have the highest earnings from private practice
- the conditions which involve the longest wait on NHS lists appear to be the mainstay of private sector workload

● the surgeons who work in the private sector are thought to have long NHS waiting lists.

Let us explore each of these coincidences in a little more detail.

The rich–poor divide

Whilst governments are sometimes reluctant to admit it (Timmins 1994), the facts suggest that health and wealth are related. Research (Townsend & Davidson 1982, Phillimore et al 1994) clearly demonstrates that it is the poorer people in any community who suffer more ill health and die earlier. Whilst a health service cannot take the sole responsibility for the variations that occur in the health of a population, it surely has the responsibility to minimize such variation and certainly has the duty not to make matters worse. The medical profession passionately believes that priority for treatment should be determined on clinical criteria and yet we find that many operations are done more frequently, and sooner, on those who can afford to pay. The question hovering over this book is whether the health service system in this country (state, voluntary and private) is compounding the problem of inequality rather than closing the gap. If the poor are less healthy than the rich, does the fact that they wait longer for treatment make matters worse or is it a cause of the rich–poor divide?

Long waits often occur in regions where there are a lot of private beds

At an early stage in work on the National Waiting List Initiative, I examined the relationship between the provision of private beds and the length of waiting lists and waiting time. At a regional level in England there did appear to be some relationship between the length of waiting time and the number of private beds available. Figure 1.6 shows that in 1989, with one or two exceptions, the regions that had the higher level of private bed provision per population were those that had the higher percentage of patients waiting over a year for treatment. Should patients be grateful that there are additional private beds in their region in order to take pressure off the NHS, or should they feel that the provision of those extra beds has resulted in the

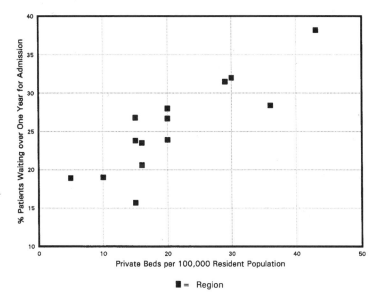

Figure 1.6   Relating private bed provision to waiting time – English RHAs 1989

Source:
House of Commons Health Committee 1991

surgeons in some regions spending more time in the private sector and allowing the NHS lists to rise?

The long-wait specialties are the main private practice specialties

It has been argued (Dean 1993) that private medicine has distorted the demand for certain specialties, because 20% of consultants carry out 66% of the private work. Publications about hospital waiting lists in England show 62 medical and surgical specialties (Department of Health, NHS Management Executive 1992). Whether specialties are ranked by the size of the waiting list or by the length of time for patients waiting, the same specialties consistently recur at the top of the list. These same specialties also have the highest private practice earnings in this country (Monopolies and Mergers Commission 1994a). Table 1.3 shows quite simply that the specialties with the longest waiting lists attract the highest private practice incomes. Is it a coincidence that the specialties that have the longest waiting times create the highest income for consultants?

Table 1.3 Specialties ranked in terms of waiting list time, size and private sector income

Specialty	Long waiting times Rank	High private practice earning Rank	Large waiting lists Rank
Trauma and orthopaedics	1	2	2
General surgery	2	6	1
Plastic surgery	3	1	8
ENT	4	3	4
Ophthalmology	5	5	5
Obstetrics and gynaecology	6	7	3
Oral surgery	7	9	7
Urology	8	4	6

Source:
Long waiting times = number of patients waiting over a year on 31 March 1992
Large waiting lists = number of in-patients and day cases on 31 March 1992
Above from DoH Waiting List In-patients and Day Cases, England at 31 March 1992
High private practice earning = Median gross earning per annum 1991–92
From Monopolies and Mergers Commission Report 'Private medical services' February 1994

The long-wait NHS conditions are the common private practice procedures

Studies of long NHS waiting lists have consistently shown that a few surgical operations take up the bulk of each specialty's waiting list. In general surgery, varicose veins and hernia operations constituted over 40% of NHS waiting lists (Davidge et al 1987) and those two operations were the most frequently occurring procedures in general surgery in the private sector in 1981, 1986 and 1992–93 (Nicholl et al 1984, Nicholl et al 1989, Williams & Nicholl 1994). In other specialties, the story was much the same. In orthopaedics, hip replacements and arthroscopies were two of the most frequent operations, whilst ENT was dominated by tonsils and adenoids, and ophthalmology by cataract surgery. Yet again, in these specialties the conditions that most frequently occur on NHS waiting lists are the 'bread and butter' of the work undertaken in independent hospitals. Is it a coincidence that the very conditions that have long NHS waiting times are those that dominate private sector activity?

Long waiting lists are sometimes associated with surgeons who do a lot of private practice

The only two books published in Britain about waiting lists (Yates 1987, Frankel & West 1993) are at pains to point out that there is little other than anecdotal evidence to support this contention. The issue has consistently been a contentious subject, but there is one small study by Ian Harvey (Frankel & West 1993) who compared two small groups of general surgeons. The first group of six surgeons undertook no private practice and the other seven did do so. Those with no private practice had an average waiting list of 111 patients, whilst those with private practice had an average waiting list of 286. Harvey argued that whilst the data had statistical significance, the small scale of the data provided only a broad indication, and did not determine any cause or effect. Whilst it appeared that private practitioners had statistically significant longer waiting lists, his conclusion was that the area was suitable for more work in order 'to raise the level of debate above the merely speculative and anecdotal'. Is it significant that this type of study is so difficult to do and is there something to hide?

Surgeons can more than double their income by undertaking private practice; 55% of consultants earn more than £20 000 on top of their £40 000 NHS salary and over 1300 of them are earning more than £100 000 on top of their NHS salary (Monopolies and Mergers Commission 1994a). These figures exclude earnings from legal fees, insurance cases, etc., and they are the declared earnings of consultants. The figures refer to all consultants, but it is the surgeons rather than the physicians who earn substantial sums from private practice. The NHS salaries alone seem very high to those in our society who are unemployed and many would wonder how additional earnings could be justified. The private sector, however, provides an extremely lucrative and financially tempting arena for the young surgeon and some senior registrars see NHS work as a 'loss-leader'. Politicians and NHS management effectively regard the additional earnings as a means of paying surgeons more money, on the grounds that a surgeon on only £40 000 per year, earns considerably less than many in senior-level posts in industry, commerce and the city.

There are many who feel that most consultants deserve to be paid as much as the chief executive of British Gas and yet he receives a pay rise that is in itself more than any top surgeon's annual NHS salary. In such circumstances, private practice becomes a form of higher income supplement. A surgeon can double his NHS income by simply operating on 2–3 private patients per week or even by just devoting each Saturday morning to seeing patients in private rooms. One of the best known commentators on private health care (Laing 1992b), when reviewing the growth in the volume of private work in the London area, raised the question of how this was being achieved by consultants 'without compromising their NHS service'. He went on to say it 'is a conundrum which has not yet been satisfactorily answered'. Why does that question remain unanswered?

These five coincidences do not provide any evidence to prove one way or another that private practice has any harmful or helpful effect on the NHS.

COINCIDENCE FUELLED BY SUSPICION?

There are other factors that worry the patient, but yet leave the professionals unconcerned. The coincidences just discussed are set alongside five other factors:

- the rapid growth and sheer size of the private sector
- the fact that surgical decision-making is not entirely a precise science
- the NHS does not supply sufficient resources to meet surgical demand
- junior surgeons do much of the operating in the NHS
- the management of medicine appears to be somewhere between difficult and impossible.

Private surgery is now big business

The private sector of 40 years ago was extremely small compared with the size of the NHS and, effectively, was simply a service for the very rich. In 1955, only 1% of the population were insured for private health care and in most small towns and

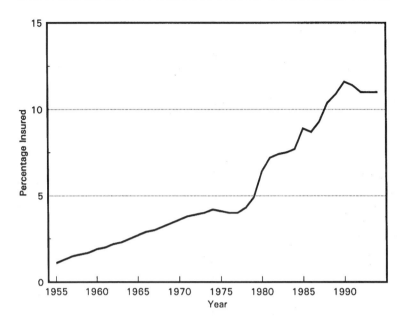

Figure 1.7   Proportion of the UK population privately insured

Source:
Laing's Review of Private Healthcare 1993

cities there were no private hospitals with an operating theatre. Private patients were treated in the NHS and were given single rooms on the end of main wards. Patients paid both the surgeon for the operation and the NHS for the accommodation. Now, private practice is big business. The proportion of the population insured for private health care has risen from 1% to 11% (*Laing's Review of Private Healthcare* 1993, Fig. 1.7). The number of private hospitals has increased from 150 in 1979 to 222 in 1994 and the number of available beds from 6671 to 11 520 in the same period.

In 1993, there were 447 private hospital operating theatres available for the use of surgeons in Britain. The volume of work that has gone through these theatres has increased. In 1981, it was estimated that 344 008 private patients were admitted per annum, but 10 years later the figure had increased to 678 703 (Nicholl et al 1984, Williams & Nicholl 1994). Any private surgery that did occur outside the NHS of 20 years ago was quite often done on Saturdays or weekday evenings, but today two-thirds of all private operations in independent hospitals take place during the working day, Monday to Friday, 9.00 a.m. to 5.00 p.m. (Laing 1992a). Private operations in the private sector and the NHS combined probably now amount to over three-quarters of a million operations per year, compared with around three million planned operations in the NHS. Private surgery is big business and it is virtually all conducted by consultants who work for the NHS. How is this achieved, given the enormous pressures within the NHS?

Surgery is not always an exact science

One of a surgeon's principle responsibilities is to decide whether or not an operation is needed, and if so, at what moment it is appropriate to undertake that operation. For some illnesses and injuries the decisions are quite straight forward and virtually all surgeons agree with each other on both the need for, and timing of, the operation. A patient arriving at an Accident and Emergency department with a broken arm would get the same response from every orthopaedic surgeon in the country – operate to repair the broken arm and do it within hours rather than days. Similarly, none of the surgeons would perform the same operation on the other unbroken arm!

But the treatment of much illness and disease is less clear cut. Arthritis in a knee joint, for example, develops over a period of years; the point at which any surgeon would choose to operate, and even opinion on whether or not the symptoms are severe enough to warrant an operation, vary from surgeon to surgeon. For most operations there are those patients for whom all would agree that the operation is appropriate and those for whom all would agree that the operation is not needed; but by far the biggest group of patients lies between these extremes. When a large proportion of operations are discretionary, are consultants tempted to place patients on waiting lists as a means of increasing waiting time and thus encouraging private patients to jump the queue?

The NHS does not supply sufficient resources to meet surgical need

Surgeons and managers have long argued that the NHS is given insufficient resources to meet the needs of an ageing population.

Enoch Powell as Minister of Health observed that (Powell 1976), 'One of the most striking features of the National Health Service is the continual, deafening chorus of complaint which rises day and night from every part of it' for more money. If we had more surgeons, and those surgeons that we do have had more resources, then we could treat more patients and waiting times would be shorter. In recent years it has been claimed that there is an increasing problem because of the closure of beds and theatres, either at the end of a financial year or as a longer term effort to 'rationalize' services, or simply to save money. In the 8 months from April to November 1993, 44% of surgical divisions were told to reduce or stop some activity (Beecham 1994a). The past few years have seen the NHS increasingly less able to provide an adequate number of operating sessions for many of its surgeons.

Junior surgeons do much of the operating

The amount of work undertaken by junior staff can vary enormously and is partly dependent on the numbers and level of experience of junior staff and the complexity or urgency of the surgery to be undertaken. It is, however, said to be common for up to half the operations in a hospital to be performed by junior surgeons. Does this mean that some consultant surgeons delegate a high proportion of their work in order to concentrate on their private practice? None of the advice offered in a consultant contract, or its surrounding regulations, mentions the division of work between juniors and seniors. The juniors take on a significant proportion of some areas of the work, especially in respect of emergency patients. There is no specific requirement for particular levels of work to be achieved by either party and, technically speaking, a consultant could delegate all his operating to a junior and not be in breach of contract. If it is true that junior surgeons in training do a substantial proportion of the work in the NHS, does it mean that the consultant who wishes to minimize his NHS workload is given every opportunity so to do?

The medical profession is powerful and difficult to 'manage'

The medical profession is a highly-qualified and well-respected group in society. Their specialized knowledge and skills in the area of illness and health leave laypersons, including managers, in awe of their professional power. We do not always understand the words they use, and yet we have a tremendous and usually deserved, trust in what they do. Politicians and managers have in the past relied heavily on their advice in determining the need for, and distribution of, resources. The work of consultants is difficult to monitor and there is little capacity for society to perform any external check on the quality and quantity of their work. Health service managers find that the measurement of clinical activity is technically very difficult and that reliable data is hard to come by, and even harder to interpret.

In recent years the medical profession has felt that their influence has been eroded, but neither patient, politician nor manager feel able to control medical decision-making. On the one hand, surgeons resent politicians and managers interfering with the priority of patients on waiting lists, when certain groups of patients on waiting lists are given Patients' Charter commitments that guarantee admission by a certain date. On the other hand, the NHS neither collects nor publishes data about the workload of individual surgeons, nor, until this year, has there been any study of the comparative workload of NHS and private sector work for individual surgeons. Why are politicians and managers so loathe to examine this subject?

Health service managers now operate in a market place which demands that they balance their accounts or lose their jobs. They are currently encouraging the growth of private facilities in NHS hospitals in order to generate income. At one stage, NHS managers even proposed a 'fast tracking' system (Anderson 1988) as a solution to reducing waiting time. There is little thought for how this might affect the equity of access for the population they serve. Hospital Trusts appear reluctant to challenge the balance between private sector activity and NHS activity and this may be because of the revenue that the hospital receives from its private patients (Fletcher 1994, Brindle 1994). Purchasing district health authorities have no right of access to data about the activity in the private sector despite the fact that over 10% of the population is insured for private health care. Does this mean that balancing the books now has priority over providing equitable access to care?

The patient is faced with five coincidences fuelled by five factors that generate suspicion, yet the total appears to convince no-one of the need for action. Together these ten factors create apprehension about the way in which the private sector and NHS work alongside each other. They do not, either individually or collectively, provide conclusive evidence of the cause of inequity in the system, but they leave many patients in considerable doubt.

IS PRIVATE SURGERY DONE AT THE EXPENSE OF THE NHS AND ITS PATIENTS?

Historically, Britain has had a health care system which has prided itself in giving equal access to all its citizens. Whilst absolute equality is an impossible dream, society should seek to avoid systematic differences that disadvantage some groups of people. Are we now faced by real inequality in the system? Is it true that access to health care is now increasingly determined by the ability of the patient to pay, more so now than at any time in the history of the NHS? The recent reforms of the NHS have introduced a type of market that is changing the delivery of health care. Will it improve access for all, or simply skew service provision even further towards those who can afford it?

Currently surgeons, and the system in which they work, are held in varying degrees of suspicion about the inequity of long waiting times. An extreme criticism is that surgeons simply manipulate waiting lists in such a way that they maximize their income from private surgery and do little for the NHS or its patients. Another criticism is that the NHS gives its surgeons inadequate theatre, bed and staff support and thus it is hardly surprising that in any spare or unused time surgeons exercise their skills in the private sector. Is there a cosy collusion between managers, surgeons and politicians? Such suspicions are countered by the view that some of the work undertaken in the private sector, often in the early morning, late evening and at week-ends, actually saves an enormous burden falling on the NHS and helps to keep waiting lists and waiting time shorter.

The patient seems ill-served by the system and neither the individual patient nor the population as a whole appears to have much in the way of a mechanism to help investigate the inequality. Consumer associations and community health councils have had little success in investigating, let alone changing, the system. The media's delight in highlighting scurrilous individual examples has done little to challenge the total system. The churches stay remarkably quiet, as the inequality in our culture grows. Inequality grows with apathy. Patients see that surgeons benefit financially from the way in which the NHS and the private sector interact. They see that surgeons have no incentive to change the system and even suspect they may deliberately make matters worse. The current system appears morally corrupt.

The claims and counter claims go back and forth. When children in a darkened room argue whether a coin has landed on its head or its tail, the simple answer is to turn on the light. If the workload of surgeons in both the public and private sectors was open to public examination, then the facts would be plain for all to see. Despite repeated requests for a full examination of both the NHS and private sector workload of each surgeon, this data remains hidden. In the absence of complete evidence this book attempts to piece together previously unpublished material with existing evidence, to examine more closely the work of surgeons and the way their work is monitored by the managers in the NHS. The rest of this book examines:

- whether there is apathy, cover-up or misplaced concern about the consultants' contract
- the degree of science in clinical decision making
- the level of consultants' operative workload within the NHS
- the amount of time consultants spend in the private sector
- the results of piecing together the evidence
- the question of what we can do to improve equality of access to health care in Britain.

A tale of two cities?

There are two cities – one where you pay to be treated and avoid waiting, the other where you don't pay, but do wait. In the first city are the rich and those in better health. They not only get quicker treatment, but quite often more treatment. The citizens are usually treated by highly trained consultant surgeons. In the second city are the poor and those more prone to ill-health. They get proportionately less care and that which they do receive is often provided by junior staff.

2

Apathy, cover-up or misplaced concern?

NO MAN CAN SERVE TWO MASTERS

The coincidences and suspicions outlined in the first chapter of this book are heightened by the nature of the consultant's contract of employment. The very use of the word contract is an anathema to the professional who regards his or her commitments to duty to be such that there is no need to specify details about hours worked or conditions of service. Professionals see themselves as totally committed to their vocation and the specification of working arrangements seems an unnecessary bureaucratic detail. Society largely respects this view, and this is reflected in the flexible nature of the contractual agreements between the government and the medical profession. Recognizing that professionals will regularly be prepared to work long hours in excess of a normal working week, the NHS has drawn up a form of contractual agreement that many would regard as being benign.

To the outsider, the level of freedom in those contracts appears unsurpassed. Within a 35-hour working week, time is allowed for travelling to work. Even consultants who work at only one hospital are allowed to claim travelling time to and from work within their contracted hours. The regulations about travelling times between hospitals can be generously interpreted. There are 2 district general hospitals, only 6 miles apart, served by 5 consultants in a single specialty, each of whom are allowed $3^1/_2$ hours per week travelling time. In total, 5 complete half-days each week are set aside for travelling, and yet, if 4 of the surgeons were simply re-allocated, 2 to each hospital, an extra 4 sessions per week of clinical activity could be achieved. In one region alone, 26 of 42 ophthalmologists had split-site contracts of this nature. The petty debates that can occur between surgeons and managers about entitlement to travelling time seem far removed from the notion of professional commitment. Such debates are not so frequently heard in discussion with the professional engineers, musicians, bankers, architects or others. They too work exceedingly long hours without any specific over-time payments, but do not usually regard travelling time as part of their working day.

The most surprising feature of the consultants' contract is that they are legally entitled to work both for the NHS and the private sector. This concept is quite foreign to the normal rules of engagement in commerce, to the guidelines offered for probity in the public sector and to the stance taken in many ethical and religious codes. It is not considered acceptable commercial prac-tice to allow a telephone engineer to exercise control over the installation of telephones in such a way that extra income could be earned by installing telephones in the evenings or at week-ends. He or she would certainly not have a contract that was flexible enough to allow the installation of telephones during the normal working day for additional personal income. Probity in the public sector demands that public officials declare any conflicts of interest and refrain from any debate or decision-making in cases where conflict occurs (House of Commons 1994). Religious teachings express the difficulty with precision and clar-ity – no servant can serve two masters (Luke 16: 13).

Does the considerable flexibility in consultants' contracts provide scope for those who might wish to short change the NHS? Even if such abuse does not occur, should not the system have some tighter specification and control to protect consul-tants from unfair criticism? The freedom allowed the medical profession could enable it to rig the market by producing artifi-cial waiting lists or simply by giving the impression that long waiting times are highly likely. This would have the effect of forcing patients to pay unnecessarily for private care and at the same time cause groups of NHS patients, who do not pay for private treatment, to wait longer than they need. How did this capacity for 'insider dealing' come about?

THE ORIGINS OF AMBIGUITY

Before the NHS was formed, consultants worked independently and often gave freely of their time to work in a voluntary capacity in hospitals. At the time of the establishment of the NHS, Aneurin Bevan, the minister responsible for drafting the NHS legislation, had had difficulty in persuading the consultants to join the new NHS. It was said that he only persuaded them to join by 'stuffing their mouths with gold' (Abel-Smith 1964). I doubt whether today's consultants, with a starting salary of about £40 000 per year, would regard that statement as having much currency.

For years the relationship between politicians and the medical profession has been delicate, with politicians fearing that to upset the consultants might mean they would leave the NHS. Politicians appear happy to allow private practice to continue as it supplements consultant incomes and saves the government revenue, as the NHS cannot afford to pay the going rate for their skills. It was in 1955 that a carefully worded agreement between the medical profession and the NHS made it clear that consultants could work for the NHS and yet still undertake private practice. The agreement, in the form a joint statement issued by the Ministry of Health and the Joint Consultants Committee, (DHSS 1979a) included the following statement:

It is recognized that some consultants, while prepared to *devote substantially the whole of their time to hospital work and to give it priority on all occasions,* would prefer a maximum part-time to a whole-time contract. Ever since 1948 it has been the Ministry's view that, subject always to the needs of the hospital service, employing Boards should in this matter take into account the circumstances and preferences of the consultants concerned.

The agreement was reaffirmed in 1961 when the Joint Consultants Committee again discussed the dual employment system with the Ministry of Health (DHSS 1979a). They reminded consultants of their obligations, pointing out that: *'Under the agreement it* (the employing authority) *can expect as much from him* (the consultant) *on a maximum part-time contract as on a whole-time contract.'*

In 1975, when Barbara Castle was Minister of Health, there were somewhat strained relations with the medical profession and the issue of opting for maximum part-time contracts again raised its head. On 17 April that year, Mrs Castle endorsed the view of the Chairman of the Central Consultants' and Specialists' Committee of 1955 (DHSS 1979a) who had said, 'The spirit of the agreement is that the difference between a maximum part-time and a whole-time consultant is not the amount of work that either does but the difference in legal relations.' Her letter (DHS 1979b) to the British Medical Association included the comment that:

It is accepted that it represented and still represents a compromise to meet the needs both of the employing authority and of the consultant. The former needs to secure substantially the whole of the consultant's professional time, and the latter accepts this obligation and that of giving priority to his NHS duties on all occasions. However, in interpreting this latter obligation I accept that it can only operate in the light of the consultant's ethical obligation to all his patients when emergencies arise. The other part of the compromise is the need of the maximum part-time consultant to enjoy – within the exercise of his professional judgment – sufficient flexibility in making arrangements to allow him to carry on private patient practice, a right to which the option entitles him (and in return for which he foregoes a part of the aggregate whole-time salary).

Subsequent changes to the contract by a Conservative government in 1979 (DHSS 1979c) now leave the vast majority of consultants on one of two contracts; either full-time or maximum part-time. A full-time contract with the NHS permits a surgeon to undertake some private practice, providing that it does not exceed 10% of his gross earnings. As the starting salary for a consultant in a full-time post is around £40 000, a ceiling of £4000 could very quickly be breached by only a modest amount of private practice. The proportion of Britain's total 20 000 consultants who have full-time NHS appointments varies between specialties. In some medical and laboratory specialties many consultants hold full-time contracts and do very little or no private practice. In anaesthetics about one-half of the consultants have full-time contracts, whereas in the surgical specialties less than one-quarter of surgeons hold a full-time contract.

The vast majority of surgeons have what is called a maximum part-time contract. This enables a consultant to earn as much private income as he wishes, provided he devotes substantially the whole of his time to the NHS. In return for this, he foregoes one-eleventh of his salary. For any manager trying to interpret the regulations, advice given about the compromise of the maximum part-time contract is in the best traditions of the comedy-sketch civil servant – it is delightfully imprecise, flexible, and ambiguous. Enshrined in the letters and circulars about contractual conditions are clauses that allow consultants to do a certain amount of private work during normal working hours – even though their time should be mainly devoted to the NHS – but with no specification about how much or how little is allowed.

CALLING FOR CLARITY

Towards the end of the 1980s, there were a number of calls for clarification of the contractual position of consultants and also for studies of the amount of work they undertake and the time they spend in the NHS and private sectors. In May 1987, the chief officers of the West Midlands Regional Health Authority were given evidence about the substantial differences between waiting times in the NHS and the private sector and of some low levels of activity within the NHS by consultants who had contracts to work in both sectors. They were told that there was no information available about the volume of work undertaken in private rooms and private hospitals and, although an examination of surgical activity was called for, none was forthcoming.

In December 1987, managers in the same region sought the advice of their Regional Medical Officer on the number of sessions that consultants might be allowed to spend on private practice during the normal working week. The advice appeared quite straightforward: 'Systematic private sector employment during the ten sessions available from Monday to Friday is totally unacceptable. I would, however, be disinclined to regard Saturday morning work in the same vein' (personal communication 1987). Trying to take action on that advice was not so easy. When the Regional Health Authority was faced with evidence of a surgeon spending 4 half-days per week in his private rooms they failed to challenge his behaviour and as a result there was no change in the surgeon's weekly pattern of work.

Other regions had more success. In the Wessex Region, the Regional Medical Officer advised that 'it is not acceptable ... to undertake a regular and planned commitment to private practice covering a full half day each week, during the normal working hours on Mondays to Fridays' (National Audit Office 1989) on a maximum part-time contract. One of the districts within the region challenged the work patterns of three consultants and succeeded in changing the under-commitment to NHS duties.

At a national level, concerns were expressed to the Department of Health, the National Audit Office and in Parliament. The work that had commenced on the National Waiting List Initiative raised the possibility of a potential link between the substantial differences in waiting times in the NHS and the private sector and the variable commitment of some surgeons to NHS sessions. In October 1988, when I was asked to bring together a team to investigate the worst waiting lists in the country, I requested permission to audit consultants whose contractual obligations were in considerable doubt. The request (personal communication 1988a) was explicitly rejected by the Department of Health (personal communication 1988b). I was told that '... the responsibility for monitoring and follow up of unsatisfactory performance at district level as lying primarily – indeed, solely – with the Regional Health Authority'. It was made quite clear there was no role for a 'private investigator'. In a letter (personal communication 1988c) 2 months later to the National Audit Office and the Department of Health I pressed the point again:

The lack of clarity regarding the NHS commitments of consultant staff and the inadequate monitoring of those commitments leaves uncertainty as to whether or not there is any abuse of NHS contracts in order to increase private practice activity. The only way to clarify this issue is to undertake direct observations of selected consultants, particularly in those sessions which do not have any specified NHS commitments. Unless you or the DHSS are prepared to initiate such studies, the question of the abuse of the NHS contractual commitment will never be satisfactorily clarified one way or the other.

The lack of response seemed to signal a determined unwillingness to examine the issue.

Dogged defence from the civil service and auditors was not reserved for outsiders like myself. Questions in the House of Commons were batted off in a masterly fashion. In November 1987 (Bottomley 1987) Mrs Virginia Bottomley, then a back bench MP, asked, 'What proposals are there to make consultants' contracts more explicit?' to which the reply came back, 'We have no plans at present to change consultant contracts.' She tried again 4 months later, (Bottomley 1988) but once again was despatched to the boundary. Even the Prime Minister, Margaret Thatcher, showed concern about the potential abuse of clinical freedom, early in 1988, but to no avail. Despite the interest in the subject within the Downing Street Policy Unit in 1988 and 1989 the issue became submerged in the discussions about reforming the NHS.

THE DAVIS–NICHOL LINE

In January 1990, two lines of enquiry coincided in an unexpected location. The Public Accounts Committee were due to discuss a report by the Comptroller and Auditor General on the NHS and independent hospitals (National Audit Office 1989). The National Audit Office had not been as unwilling to examine the subject, as I had at first expected. Their report set out to examine two issues. First, did the NHS make effective use of the facilities offered by the independent sector? Secondly, were satisfactory arrangements in place to ensure that consultants fulfilled their NHS commitments? Whilst members of the Public Accounts Committee were studying their report, one of the members, a Birmingham MP, received information about the private Priory Hospital in Edgbaston, Birmingham.

The Priory Hospital produced a booklet for general practitioners which listed the clinical facilities available at that hospital. There were 178 hospital consultant users, and for each consultant appeared an address, which was either an NHS hospital, a private hospital or private consulting rooms. Also listed were 87 consultants who held out-patient consultation sessions at the Hospital. For a handful of the consultants specific clinic times were not given, but merely a note that appointments were available at 'variable times'. The majority, however, had routine out-patient clinics listed as being held at the hospital. The sessions for these clinics varied in length between 1 and 7 hours and the hospital held 51 full clinics and 19 half clinics during the normal working week. A further 19 sessions were held in evenings or on Saturday mornings. The precise NHS contractual position of each of the consultants was not published in the Priory Hospital document, although it was subsequently independently confirmed that, at least, 10 consultants had full-time NHS contracts and that the vast majority of the remainder were on maximum part-time contracts.

Of the 10 consultants with full-time contracts, 2 were specified as having consultations at variable times, 2 were listed as having times that overlapped with part of the working day and the remaining 6 were listed as having full half-day sessions in the private hospital. For the remaining consultants who had a maximum part-time contract (or, in one or two cases, a part-time contract) some undertook clinics outside normal hours or did not have specified times for clinics at all; but some undertook one, two or even three half-day clinics in the Priory Hospital.

The ready availability of consultation time during the working day at the Priory Hospital contrasted with a statement quoted in the Comptroller and Auditor General's report, in which a regional medical advisor had said, 'it is not acceptable ... to undertake a regular and planned commitment to private practice covering a full half-day each week, during the normal working hours on Monday to Fridays' as a maximum part-time consultant (National Audit Office 1989). It was this contrast that provoked some discussion in the Public Accounts Committee on 22 January 1990 when a most remarkable exchange took place (House of Commons Committee of Public Accounts 1990). After all the compromise and ambiguity, a straight question was met with a straight answer. Terry Davis MP asked, 'How many half days would it be unreasonable for a consultant to take off for private practice if he is full-time or maximum part-time?' The Chief Executive of the NHS who was its accounting officer to Parliament replied, 'It certainly would not be more than one.' For the first time in the history of the NHS there was, at a national level, a guideline that managers and consultants could understand.

In case there was any ambiguity, 1 month later the Chief Executive, (now Sir), Duncan Nichol wrote to each of the regional Chief Executives re-stating his reply to the Public Accounts Committee. The reply was clearly understood, but not liked by the Hospital Consultants and Specialists Association and in response to their enquiries Duncan Nichol (personal communication undated) again spelt out the interpretation:

At the hearing before the Commons Public Accounts Committee in January, a number of questions were raised about the private work of NHS consultants. I said, and repeated in my letter of 20th February, that I took the view that, particularly for those on maximum part-time contracts, one *planned* private session a week might be acceptable, but where two or more *planned* sessions were undertaken privately, such an arrangement would be unacceptable. Where a consultant had two planned sessions in a private hospital there would be a conflict with his commitment to accord priority at all times to his NHS work. Cases may need to be considered individually, but I would find it difficult to accept that any consultants, whether whole-time or maximum part-time, who undertook two or more planned private sessions could be said to be fulfilling their contractual commitments to the NHS.

The Public Accounts Committee and the wider public were further assured that the planned changes of placing consultant contracts at a local level and the introduction of consultant job plans would now permit closer monitoring of any potential problem. It appeared that there was no longer a problem and, as a Department of Health spokesman assured *The Times* (Sherman 1990): 'Under the new arrangements it should be much easier to find out if they [the consultants] are sticking to their contracts.' The Committee was not so sure, and in its formal report (House of Commons Committee of Public Accounts 1990) it included two recommendations which expressed their reservations:

The introduction of more precise job plans for consultants is a step in the right direction; but we emphasize that, to be effective, these will require firm management but at the same time should not burden consultants with unnecessary bureaucracy; we note that job plans will not give health authorities a view of consultants' total National Health Service and private commitments. We believe that health authorities need a more accurate picture of the total level of consultants' commitments to ensure that their responsibilities for the treatment of patients are not put in jeopardy through working excessive hours.

The Department responded by commenting that 'health authorities have only an indirect interest in the work which consultants may do outside the NHS' and that the newly agreed 'job plans will strengthen the ability of NHS managers to ensure that consultants are fulfilling their NHS duties'(Financial Secretary to the Treasury 1990).

The debate in the Public Accounts Committee led to an enquiry in the West Midlands about the situation at the Priory Hospital. The West Midlands Regional Health Authority initiated an enquiry into the 87 consultants listed by the hospital. It emerged that 2 of the consultants were actually a dietitian and a speech therapist, 4 were not employed as consultants by the West Midlands Regional Health Authority, 9 had retired and 3 held only honorary contracts with the Health Authority. Of the remaining 69 consultants, only 49 had fixed sessions listed at the Priory Hospital during normal working hours. The Regional Health Authority, strengthened by the debate held in the Public

Accounts Committee, took the view that full-time consultants would not be expected to hold regular fixed sessions within normal working hours and that consultants on maximum part-time contracts would reasonably be allowed one half-day private practice session during the working week.

Using those criteria, the Health Authority decided that 29 maximum part-time consultants, who had only one fixed session scheduled at the Priory Hospital, should not be investigated. It is interesting to note the extremely narrow terms of reference chosen by the Health Authority. At no point did it check whether any of these 29 consultants were surgeons who might also operate during the working day, neither did they check whether any of the 29 consultants worked in other private hospitals or rooms during the normal working week. Instead, they decided to review the position of only 19 consultants, 8 of whom held maximum part-time contracts and 11 of whom were full-time. The enquiry was further reduced from 19 to 17 in view of the retirement of one consultant and the fact that another was gravely ill at the time of the enquiry. The method of enquiry was then to write to each of the consultants concerned and, where appropriate, discuss the matter with the consultant directly. No study was made of actual working hours at the Priory Hospital or any other private hospital, nor was any study undertaken on the operating time of consultant surgeons. The enquiry consisted mainly of a debate between managers and surgeons about the consulting times listed at the Priory Hospital.

Two points emerged from the study. First, it was argued that there was a distinction to be made between the availability of consulting time, as listed by the Priory Hospital directory, and the actual attendance at the private hospital by the consultants concerned. It was pointed out that consultants did not necessarily attend each week at the times specified by the Priory Hospital. The second point was that the consultants claimed that they worked long hours in the NHS that were well in excess of their formal contractual position. In every case it was argued that although private work was done at the Priory Hospital, it was never done to the detriment of the NHS.

Two of the consultants converted their contract from full-time to maximum part-time in the time between the publication of the Priory document and the enquiry. The enquiry stated (letter 1991): 'No instance had been found where private commitments were undertaken to the detriment of the NHS, which in fact, benefits from a significantly greater commitment by consultants than their formal contractual obligations would require.' The conclusions of the enquiry came as no surprise since the methodology used could not possibly have ascertained whether or not there was any detriment to the NHS. There was no data-gathering about activities at the Priory Hospital or any other private hospital which would enable the enquiry to come to such a conclusion.

AFTER THE DAVIS–NICHOL LINE

Despite the assurances from the civil service that all was now under control, the evidence gained from studying England's longest hospital waiting lists suggested that managers had no more control over the situation than they had had previously. Ministers, civil servants and auditors continued to ignore pressure from various directions to study the workload in the two sectors. The newly formed Health Committee attempted to explore the impact of private practice on waiting lists and in their first report (House of Commons Health Committee 1991) recommended:

... that the Department of Health carry out a study ... to try and determine the influence, either positive or negative, that private practice in the same unit or specialty has on the waiting list and waiting time for treatment. The results of such a survey should help inform districts in their local discussion of consultants job plans.

Later that year, another committee (House of Commons Welsh Affairs Committee 1991) undertook a similar enquiry and said:

We agree with the Health Committee that the influence of private practice be examined. Statistics about the number and type of operations carried out privately [both those with and those without medical insurance], and by whom, should be collected. Such information on private practice is necessary to identify gaps and to guide health authorities in providing for future requirements. Moreover, such information would assist management in ensuring that private practice does not interfere with the performance of the NHS.

The negative response received by the Public Accounts Committee also awaited the other select committees. The Health Committee was told by the Department of Health (Department of Health 1991):

It is not clear what would be achieved by such a study. It is of course important that Districts have a firm management grip on the work consultants do. That is best achieved by matching their service contracts to their consultants' job plans and ensuring that both are operating properly. Management is also responsible for ensuring that private practice does not, to a significant extent, interfere with the performance of the function of the health service or disadvantage non-paying patients. This is a statutory requirement and the main principle agreed with the medical profession governing the conduct of private practice in health service hospitals.

In 1990, further changes were made that helped make a tighter definition of contractual responsibilities. The government intro-duced the concept of 'job plans' (Department of Health 1990) which it was said would make the monitoring of contract compli-ance easier for managers. The job plan requires each consultant to specify for 5, 6 or 7 half-days (of the 10 half-days between Monday morning and Friday afternoon) what he or she would be doing in the NHS. For surgeons these job plan half-days are nearly always specified as being spent in the operating theatre or out-patient clinic. Subsequent examination of the introduction of job plans by the Audit Commission and the National Audit Office has shown that in many hospitals they are only a paper exercise, resented by surgeons and given scant attention by managers.

Pressure also came from outside Parliament, but one wonders whether the media might have been wiser to save their print. The *Health Service Journal* (Editorial 1992) commented on signs of panic in the world of private insurance and said:

Evidence about private medicine's impact on the length of NHS waiting lists is poor, consisting mainly of anecdotes and lacking hard facts. To argue that all private healthcare relieves the NHS of a burden it would otherwise have to shoulder is to make several large assumptions.

Is all private work done only in non-NHS time? Are NHS instruments never borrowed without permission? Are all fees from private work declared to the NHS – or to the Inland Revenue? The national Confidential Enquiry into Perioperative Deaths has highlighted the practice of junior doctors carrying out unsupervised procedures for which they are inadequately experienced; how many are unsupervised because their consultants have over-run at their private clinics?

... it is time for a proper survey into the volume of surgery done in the private sector.

In October of the following year, *The Independent* (Editorial 1993) in an even more aggressive vein suggested that:

An inquiry by the Audit Commission or the National Audit Office should be ordered. The investigation should go to the heart of why some doctors are failing to treat a sufficient number of patients. It would be independent enough to challenge consultants and government and would reveal the true story behind the delays that are costing lives.

The call for clarity continued unabated. A consumer organiza-tion recently attempted to establish how much time consultants could spend on private practice and asked the BMA for its view on the advice offered by Sir Duncan Nichol. The response was quite simple. The BMA argued that Sir Duncan was factually wrong, he had spoken out of turn and, apparently, had subse-quently been reprimanded for what he had said. Although his comments have not been formally retracted, the BMA argued that consultants can, indeed, spend 2 or more half-days of the working week in the private sector. This can be done in the 'uncommitted' sessions that are not scheduled as operating theatre or out-patient clinic time, and which are often in lieu of work done out of hours and on-call commitments.

The same response met the auditors of both the National Audit Office and the Audit Commission. The response was not, however, restricted to the BMA, but also came from the Department of Health. The Department now claims that chief executives throughout the NHS may not be aware of Sir Duncan's letter and that, in any case, it expressed a personal view which was not therefore government policy. It is quite a remarkable way of being economical with the truth. It says that letters formally sent from the Chief Executive's office may not be known about in the NHS and that the Chief Accounting Officer of the NHS only expressed a personal view when answering questions posed by the Public Accounts Committee. The change in tone is exemplified by the reaction of the DHSS to an early draft of the Audit Commission on the subject of probity in the NHS (The Audit Commission 1994a). The firm advice offered by the Audit Commission was that the NHS had:

... made its expectations of consultants very clear, and Chief Executives should ensure compliance with the guidance set out in the Chief Executive's letter of July 1990: namely, that consultants on a full-time NHS contract would not be expected to supplement their NHS salaries by more than ten per cent from private work, and that consultants under a maximum part-time contract should not devote more than one session during the normal working week to private practice.

The advice offered in the final report (The Audit Commission 1994b) was watered down and advised that:

Trusts now hold consultants' contracts and Chief Executives and Clinical Directors should therefore ensure compliance with all fixed session commitments. Job plans should be signed by two parties and reviewed annually.

The irony is that the job plans created by the Department of Health to ensure a more rigorous monitoring of contract compliance have in fact given consultants even greater freedom. The NHS and civil servants now regard the advice of Duncan Nichol as extinct. It was an erroneous personal view, which in any case was issued prior to the recent NHS reforms and contractual matters are now in the hands of Trusts.

The Department of Health no longer has any interest in, or responsibility for, what consultants do at a local level. The Davis–Nichol line simply does not apply. Consultants can indeed spend 2, 3 or even 4 half-days per week working in the private sector and yet, apparently, still devote substantially the whole of their time to the NHS.

SO WHY NO ENQUIRY?

This chapter started by asking whether there was apathy, cover-up or misplaced concern about the consultant contract. For 8 years I have been calling for clarity about the terms of consultant contracts and for an enquiry about the actual workings of the contract. I have received enthusiastic support from three parliamentary select committees and many journalists and had some hesitant interest from the National Audit Office and the Audit Commission. I have encountered disinterest and defensiveness from managers and surgeons and faced disinterest and outright hostility from the Department of Health's ministers and civil servants. There seem to be three possible explanations for the lack of a study into this issue.

1. Apathy – there is a problem, but it is difficult to handle and people are slow to take action.
2. Cover-up – there is a problem and vested interests ensure the status quo remains unchanged.
3. Misplaced concern – there is no problem.

Apathy

Perhaps, initially, those responsible were simply not aware of any pressure to examine the issue and only recently have been persuaded that there is a problem. Whilst all the parties concerned genuinely want to address the issue, they find it difficult to coordinate their efforts. As individual groups they are less sure of their ground. Surgeons are reluctant to take action against their fellow professionals and any individual case of abuse of contract is only apparent to a small group of immediate colleagues. There is no easy mechanism available and few guidelines. Taking action against friends and colleagues is quite naturally put off as long as is reasonably possible. No-one wants to offend close colleagues if it can be avoided, and certainly not if there is the slightest doubt, either about the 'offence' or about the regulations. Some politicians, managers and civil servants are in awe of the medical profession and fear that they will either lose the profession from the NHS, or that an enquiry might perhaps upset the profession so badly that the amount of work undertaken in the NHS will actually decrease. The consultants increasingly feel they have lost their power base to the combined forces of politicians and managers and anyway one can hardly expect the medical fraternity itself to have much incentive to address the issues concerned.

Each of the non-medical groups involved are unsure of their responsibilities and have the additional problem of a lack of continuity amongst senior decision-makers. There are frequent changes in personnel who become like ships that pass in the night. NHS managers, who have always moved posts regularly, now do so with increasing frequency following the introduction of short-term contracts. Their roles constantly change as the structure of the NHS alters with increasing frequency. The managers appear to have more concern about the framework of the NHS than for the health status of the people they are supposed to serve. They intermingle with civil servants who are not even guaranteed to be in the same government department for any length of time. The civil servants become more fearful of taking firm stances on any subject in the face of growing job insecurity. They are like chameleons, changing their style to blend in with the latest political, ideological, academic and managerial fashions. Politicians, especially ministers, come and go, rarely last for more than 2 years at a time and soon fade from memory. Their diaries and writings sound like the books of old testament prophets (e.g. the books of Enoch and David) (Powell 1976, Owen 1976). They can be taken off the shelves occasionally, but they hardly leave a lasting impression, let alone a lasting achievement.

Arguably the most independent and, theoretically, the most secure group are the auditors of the National Audit Office and the Audit Commission. They are cautious by nature and somewhat anonymous as far as the general public and health service professionals are concerned. However, they may not have the necessary expertise to deal successfully with clinicians and at times are very sensitive to political correctness. The existence of two separate audit bodies is somewhat confusing and the two groups can appear to be vying for attention with their increasingly glossy reports. Both have recently ventured into the area of consultant contracts, but it is disappointing that it has taken them so long.

Perhaps the fact that so many different groups are involved has led each to be apathetic towards any problems that exist.

COVER-UP

Maybe these groups have something to hide. Civil servants have long been tarred with the brush of being 'economical with the truth' (Shrimsley 1994) and they are also skilled at using the 'corporate lie'. For years I have impressed on the Department of Health the need to study consultants' workload in the NHS and the private sector. When questioned about this by a journalist, 'a DoH spokesman said that the department was not aware of Mr Yates' request for such a study and none was planned' (Byrne 1991). Given the frequent letters, reports and articles on the subject, the spokesperson was either being deliberately misleading or, conveniently, was a junior selected to comment because of their ignorance of the subject. Such spokespersons can honestly say that they have heard of no such request, even though their colleagues have frequently engaged in conversations and correspondence on the same subject.

It is easy to understand that civil servants will be both 'economical with the truth' and 'economical with the action' if they are trying to maintain the status quo, but why should all the other groups be so reticent to have an enquiry? Is there some form of cover-up because the decision-makers have an undeclared interest? Many of those who have contributed to changes in health policy, including politicians, civil servants, managers, health authority chairmen and academics, have private health insurance or pay privately for treatment. In the period when the latest health reforms were being considered, both the Prime Minister and a Secretary of State for Health used private hospitals. Civil service and management professional bodies and trade unions have private schemes as do some universities, even for staff in units that study NHS management. In a bizarre twist, the Chief Executive of the NHS who at one time had taken a firm line on consultant contracts, took up a paid post within the private medical sector within a few months of leaving the NHS (Chadda 1994b).

The wealth of these decision-makers enables them to exercise a choice which others do not have. The eloquence of claiming freedom of choice ignores the fact that their ability to be seen quickly, and by a chosen consultant, is at someone else's expense. Their ability to be seen has been based on their ability to pay and not on their clinical need. The patient and the surgeon pretend that as the two systems (the NHS and the private sector) are separate, there is no need to look at how choices made in one sector might affect choices in the other. But perhaps these views are too cynical. There surely cannot be such a conspiracy from so many disparate groups.

Misplaced concern

Perhaps despite the pressure to examine the issue, there is no need to establish an enquiry. On the basis of information not available to those calling for an enquiry, the Department of Health has examined the issue and made a positive decision to take no action. In order to avoid an unnecessary debate, the evidence on which the decision was made has not been published. There is, of course, a small amount of abuse, a fact readily admitted by the medical profession itself (Lewis 1981). The occasional rotten apple, well known to the profession, must be dealt with by the consultants themselves (Vallance-Owen 1994) and in a manner which will not engender unjustified criticism of the whole profession.

It is well documented (Monopolies and Mergers Commission

1994a) that consultants work considerably more hours in the NHS than they are contracted to do and any examination of the issue will only be to the detriment of the NHS. The implication that there is any impropriety is clearly unfounded. The Church of England and, in particular, the Roman Catholic Church both work hand in hand with consultants who mix private and NHS medicine in church-owned hospitals. Neither church is knowingly going to condone an immoral or unjustified system.

We are dealing with different groups of highly professional surgeons, managers, civil servants and auditors. All are steeped in high moral values and ethics. The surgeons are members of the Royal College of Surgeons whose motto is 'Skills for the benefit of all men'. The managers, auditors and civil servants work in a country whose government has in the past had an honourable tradition of public service probity. The checks and balances in such a complex system simply could not be flouted in a way that leaves at any disadvantage the very patients they all serve.

So which explanation can we believe? All three lack evidence to support their case. If there is evidence, it is not available to the public gaze. This book tries to uncover some of the facts needed to make a judgement on whether or not the NHS and its patients are best served by a system which allows consultants to work for both the NHS and the private sector.

A tale of two cities?
Both cities are in the same kingdom, share the same government, the same civil servants and the same surgeons. The cities are controlled by people who don't want to see the separate health care systems changed. It is often the private hospitals of the first city that are used by the key decision-makers who defend the status quo.

3

SCIENCE AND DISCRETION

SURGICAL DISCRETION

Politicians and health service managers are regarded by many with a certain degree of mistrust and suspicion. The medical profession, on the other hand, has a very different public image. The vast majority of people, quite reasonably, have enormous faith in the science of medicine and in doctors. Before examining what surgeons actually do in the NHS and the private sector, it is worth considering why we so readily trust the medical profession. Our trust is based partly on the individual doctor that we meet, and partly on the scientific knowledge that he or she and the profession have. Those of us who are not medically trained assume that clinical decisions are based on detailed scientific knowledge. We accept that in the early development of techniques this might not always be the case, and realize that some experimentation is necessary for medicine to move forward. However, in the main, our ignorance contains the act of faith that medical knowledge is soundly based on science. If any problem requires surgical intervention then we expect an appropriately trained surgeon to undertake that task.

Part of the decision-making process about whether to and when to operate is based on scientific knowledge and incontrovertible facts. Each year millions of difficult operations are performed with a high rate of success. The population benefits from a reduction in pain, thanks to replacement hip joints; vastly improved eyesight as a result of cataract removal; and longer life as a result of complex heart surgery and many other operations. None of these could possibly be performed by those of us without medical training and there are few, or no, alternative cures available. There remains, however, a great deal that the scientific and medical community does not know about the causes and development of diseases. As a consequence, doctors are not always precisely sure about how to cure some diseases. Even where a medicine or a surgical operation is known to be beneficial, doctors are not always sure when to intervene. Some of the decisions that have to be made are not based on precise scientific fact.

Newton, who discovered the law of gravity, tells us that an apple will fall with an acceleration rate of 32 feet per second per second. It does not matter what size or colour of apple has dropped, it will always fall and always with the same acceleration. We accept that as an incontrovertible scientific fact. In some areas of medicine there are few scientific facts. If you have varicose veins on your legs, you will find that the surgeons who are trained to operate on such conditions have different opinions, but few facts. They will disagree about whether or not the leg should be operated on, and if the decision is to operate, whether it should be done now or later. Different forms of treatment and operation are available to the surgeons and in each case there will be varying degrees of success and different rates of recurrence of the problem. The variations are, in part, dependent on the surgeon and patient involved. Anyone who makes a study of surgical literature soon finds that surgery is not always an exact science. This chapter is not a critique of ignorance, nor a criticism of ignorance. It merely sets out to describe the extent of discretion there is for some medical and surgical decisions. It provides a context in which we can later examine the activity of surgeons in the NHS and private sector.

ONE OF THE MOST COMMON OPERATIONS

The removal of tonsils and adenoids has been one of the most common operations ever performed in the Western world. At one time, earlier in this century, it was calculated that one-third of all operations under general anaesthesia in the United States of America was the tonsils and adenoids operation (Glover 1938).

No-one would dream of having their tonsils removed by anyone other than an competent otorhinolaryngologist. The word 'oto-rhino-laryngologist' comes from the Latin for 'ear', 'nose' and 'throat' and it is used as a formal title for a group of surgeons who specialize in treating those parts of the head and neck. In the NHS they are known simply as ENT surgeons. They perform a wide range of operations including the very complex surgery described by actor Nigel Havers. As a 19-year-old he had developed a large lump in his throat which was a growth wrapped around his thyroid gland and vocal chords. He was referred to an immaculately dressed and dapper ENT surgeon, who terrified him by explaining that he was going to cut out the lump and added, 'If it is malignant, we will have to cut out everything around it, and if it is in your vocal chords they will have to go.' The lump turned out to be benign, but the operation took 8 hours (Havers & Danziger 1994). This type of complex major operation is, fortunately, quite rare and the bulk of ENT surgeons' work comprises much less major surgery.

In the early days of ENT surgery there was much dispute about the need for the removal of tonsils and adenoids despite it being the most common operation performed by ENT surgeons. In 1934 American doctors studied a group of 1000 New York schoolchildren (American Child Health Association 1934). They found that 60% of them had already had their tonsils removed. The remaining 40% were referred to a group of school doctors for a 'second opinion'. When these children were examined just under half of them were considered in need of having their tonsils removed. Those children not in need of the operation were then sent to a second group of doctors and, once again, just under half those children were thought to be in need of the operation. A third team of doctors were then asked to examine the remaining children and by the time three successive 'second opinions' had been sought, only 67 of 1000 children were spared the recommendation for a tonsillectomy operation. What scientific criteria were American school doctors using to decide whether or not a child's tonsils should be removed?

In England there is no evidence of any greater consistency in medical knowledge on the subject. In 1938, Dr J. A. Glover delivered a lecture to the Royal Society of Medicine in which he described enormous differences in the rate at which schoolchildren were admitted to hospital for tonsils operations (Glover

1938). He found that the average tonsillectomy rate for elementary schoolchildren in 1936 was 1.7%, but he was surprised to find that some local authorities had 3 times the average rate and others had less than a third of the average rate. Children were 10 times more likely to have their tonsils removed in Peterborough than they were in Hornsey, Wood Green or Finchley. He produced large coloured maps of England and Wales which showed that the extreme variations bore no relationship to environment, overcrowding, poverty, bad housing, climate, efficiency of school medical services or to any other recognizable factor. These variations usually remained consistent over the years from 1930 to 1936, but very occasionally he found a sudden change in rates. In Hornsey and Derbyshire he traced a sudden reduction in rates to the appointment of new school medical officers of health, who had used much stricter criteria in the referral of children for tonsils operations. His conclusion was that the differences could be explained not by actual medical need, but by differences in professional judgement.

Despite the warnings of Glover and others, the schools medical services in England and Wales continued to do a sterling job in referring young children for tonsillectomy. In the 1950s whole classes of schoolchildren in the Black Country would be admitted 'en block' for the operation. Perhaps the logic was that the fear of being admitted to hospitals would be less if you went with your classmates for a school trip which would include the opportunity after the operation of having ice cream. Some fifty-year-olds can still vividly remember which friends they were admitted with. All I can remember is the ice cream!

In 1972, leading ENT surgeons and child health specialists still admitted that scientific knowledge in this area was far from complete. Mawson and Stroud (1972) stated: 'In the present state of our knowledge the wisest approach to the question whether or not to remove tonsils and adenoids, especially in the very young children, is from a position of preferential conservancy. The precise immunological role of the tonsils and adenoids is still under investigation.' In simple language, they did not know what tonsils did or what they were for. Commenting on the huge ENT waiting lists that were packed with children waiting for tonsillectomies they suggested: 'It cannot be said that a waiting list in these cases is an entirely bad thing. Time alone will remove many children from the waiting list because they will grow out of their troubles.'

It was at this time, whilst working with Dr Ben Wood, a paediatrician, that I first realized that scientific precision in medicine might not be all that it seemed. We shared a concern about the length of the tonsils waiting list in a specialist children's hospital. Along with his ENT surgical colleagues, Dr Wood set up a study of the criteria used by doctors when deciding whether or not a child's tonsils and adenoids should be removed (Wood et al 1972). He argued that in Britain there would be general agreement between most doctors that a certain group of children (those who suffered chronic quinsy and those who had grossly enlarged tonsils and adenoids that were causing obstructive symptoms) should definitely have their tonsils and adenoids removed. There was a further group who might have persistent or relapsing deafness who would need adenoids removed. The remaining children were referred for less well defined reasons '... such as recurrent sore throats, frequent colds, general ill-health or abnormal tonsillar appearances. Here the need for an operation is still a matter of opinion.'

In order to explore this question further, six paediatricians examined a group of 217 children on the 'routine' ENT waiting list. These children had been listed by ENT surgeons for operation, but were not classified as being in urgent need of the operations for the type of conditions described above. They had been waiting for up to 3, sometimes 5, years for the operation. The doctors made detailed notes of each child's history and symptoms and physically examined their throats and ears. After discussions with the child's parents and the surgeon, each child was allocated to one of three groups:

- discharge as the child no longer needed the operation
- operate
- observe (i.e. bring back to the out-patient clinic at a later date to see whether or not the symptoms have changed sufficiently to either discharge the child or decide to operate).

After examination the children fell into roughly three equal groups, and only 81 had the adeno-tonsillectomy operation at that point. After 2 years the 'observe' group were seen again and once more classified as either fit for discharge, in need of the operation or to continue under observation. By the end of the study only 118 of the 217 patients had undergone the operation for which they were originally listed. It did not create much confidence in scientific medicine to think that 99 of 217 children listed for an operation turned out not to need that operation. Moreover, the 217 children studied were only a proportion of those who were invited to attend. Letters had been sent to a further 74 patients who failed to reply. Most of these had changed their minds about the need for an operation, and the conclusion was that well over half the children originally listed to have an operation were unlikely to have needed it.

A further disturbing aspect of the study was the differing results of the doctors' examination of the clinical state of the tonsils. At a joint meeting of ENT surgeons, paediatricians and general practitioners, 41 doctors were shown 9 colour slides of children's tonsils. The audience was given the choice of 'discharge', 'observe' or 'operate'. To check the consistency of individual doctors' decisions, and without their knowledge, 2 slides were shown twice. Although the doctors made decisions about 9 slides, there were actually only 7 patients' tonsils on display. The results of comparing 4 slides of the same 2 children showed that only 7 doctors made the same decisions about both patients. Different decisions about both patients were made by 15 doctors, and the rest made different decisions about one of the patients. Given that all these doctors were well used to examining tonsils, 'the value of a single inspection of the fauces [short passage between the back of the mouth and the pharynx] to decide the fate of the tonsils is shown in its true light'. The study concluded that the appearance of the tonsils was of no value in deciding whether or not to remove them. It finished by offering the advice that operations should only be performed on children who had 5 or more sore throats and more than 3 weeks off school per year and no improvement in general health. Such criteria rely heavily on parental and school attitude to illness and can hardly be classified as scientific.

It might be worth reminding ourselves that we are discussing the most commonly undertaken ENT operation of all time. In the mid-1960s it constituted two-thirds of all ENT operations. In the 1970s, 16% of all children had had the operation by the age of seven (Davie et al 1972). Both in Britain and America, Finkel (1988) estimated that two-thirds of the tonsillectomies performed need not have been undertaken. He describes this operation as 'discretionary surgery'. Even though the tonsillectomy is less 'fashionable', it is important to emphasize that the operation is still ENT's most common operation, it often dominates ENT waiting lists (Davidge et al 1987), and in recent years is increasing in frequency.

It is over 50 years since Dr Glover graphically told the story of huge variations in tonsillectomy rates from district to district across this country. I would have enjoyed sitting in the Royal Society of Medicine audience when he displayed the two colourful maps, which revealed no discernible pattern or explanation for those different rates. As I read his paper I suspected that he would have been envious of the way today's researchers can use a small microcomputer to display variations district by district, in colour, on a screen. I was drawn to my computer and looked up the 1991 data. It displayed huge variations district by district and in the previous 10 years each district has retained its place in the hierarchy. Just as Glover had found, districts with high rates in one year remained high year after year, and those with low rates remained low. As I looked at the 1991 distribution curiosity got the better of me – what was Peterborough's position? Just as in 1938, it had one of the highest rates in the country for admitting children with tonsillitis (Fig. 3.1). Would Glover have been

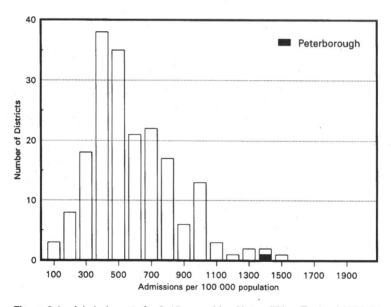

Figure 3.1   Admission rate for 0–15-year-olds with tonsillitis – England 1990–91
Source:
Department of Health HSIs 1990–91

disappointed that we have added little, if anything, to our scientific knowledge about the decision to undertake the tonsillectomy operation? All we have learnt to do is analyse more quickly the type of data that he had so painstakingly assembled.

In summary, we have in the adeno-tonsillectomy an operation which has been the subject of clinical fashion over the years. It is regarded as largely 'discretionary' judging by the huge variation there is from place to place, and for which scientific advice is, at best, unclear. And yet this is the most common operation in the ENT specialty, still representing a third of all operations carried out.

HOW MUCH SURGERY IS UNNECESSARY?

Should it be construed as a challenge to clinical freedom to ask for scientific evidence that an operation is effective? It does not seem unreasonable to ask questions about one of the most commonly performed operations of all time. In the absence of scientific knowledge and given the apparent willingness of some surgeons to follow fashion without rigorous scientific questioning, there will always remain doubts about any clinical decision to operate in a situation where symptoms are known to improve over time.

Have I been unfair in choosing the tonsils and adenoids operation to open a discussion on science and surgery? You would not think so judging by the sensational headlines in *The Sunday Times* on 27 November 1994 which said, 'Doctors claim that three in four operations are unnecessary.' It described scalpel-happy surgeons who are 20 times more likely to operate than some of their colleagues, and commented that millions of pounds were spent each year on operations that are of questionable value (Rogers 1994). The apparently scurrilous headlines were based on a leaked draft of a serious academic work which was studying variations in clinical practice over very many years. The research report, commissioned by the Department of Health, was due to be published in the spring of 1995, but it is unlikely to contain such eye-catching phrases.

The fact is that the actual procedure involved in each surgical operation is, in most cases, safe and effective. The problem is more frequently whether or not surgeons are choosing the right patients to operate on and whether or not they are doing the operation at the right time. We cannot take an over-simplistic view which simply categorizes certain operations as successful, totally ineffective or dangerous. The argument about the tonsillectomy operation is not that it is never appropriate – the argument is about which patients it should be performed on and at what stage.

Surgical procedures are usually classed as diagnostic or therapeutic. Diagnostic procedures find out what is wrong with us and therapeutic operations try to improve our health by removing, repairing, replacing or reshaping parts of our bodies. The removal of cataracts and replacement of hip joints are two examples of highly effective operations which are judged as such by patients, scientists, surgeons and even accountants. Whilst surgical history is littered with examples of failed operations (Bunker et al 1977) it is more appropriate to examine the profile (Fig. 3.2) of each operation in order to understand how valuable that operation might be, and to how many patients. We need to identify how much scientific evidence is available for each operation

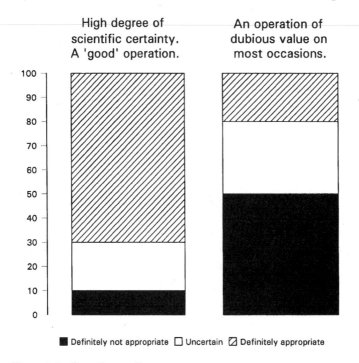

Figure 3.2   Operation profiles

which will help us complete an appropriate profile. One leading scientific surgeon, who has done much to persuade the Royal College of Surgeons to invest considerable time and effort in surgical audit is Mr Brendan Devlin. Author of dozens of scientific papers, he campaigns under the banner: 'All free health care must be effective'. He, and many others, point out that the likelihood of being referred or admitted to hospital depends as much on the opinions of doctors as it does on the condition of the patient (Bevan & Devlin 1994).

The huge variations in admission rates for tonsillectomy shown in Figure 3.1 occur in many other conditions, whether you examine GP referral rates, operation rates or surgical admission rates. In all areas it is common to find a three- or fourfold variation in rates. These variations are made greater by the uncertainty and ignorance of the outcome of many surgical interventions. Whilst new drugs are thoroughly tested before being introduced, there is no such requirement to test and prove new surgical procedures.

TOP OPERATIONS?

The National Health Service attempts to record every operation undertaken in an NHS hospital. Year on year it records more operations and by 1992–93 it achieved 5.1 million operations per year. To be technical, they are not operations, but 'surgical procedures'. Some of the procedures listed are not what members of the public would have classified as an operation. Over half a million are associated with pregnancy and childbirth and more than one million others relate to terminations of pregnancy, sterilizations, transfusions, injections and diagnostic procedures. Keeping track of over five million operations per year is no mean task. Each operation is given a code determined by the Office of Population Censuses and Surveys (OPCS) (OPCS 1990). The OPCS have produced a list of over 4000 separate surgical procedures. To try and simplify the analysis they group the procedures into a set of about 1000 operation types. Each group includes a set of similar operations and, in many cases, the group is dominated by one main operation, with a few similar operations included.

Table 3.1 lists 10 of the most common procedures undertaken in the NHS and they alone represent over a quarter of all

Table 3.1   Ten common operations

Common name of operation	OPCS code	Number of operations 1992–93
1. Endoscopy (upper gastrointestinal tract)	G45	299 686
2. Group including termination of pregnancy	Q11	152 962
3. Cystoscopy	M45	152 130
4. Dilatation and curettage (D&C) (and others)	Q10	126 636
5. Extraction of teeth (especially wisdom)	F09	93 052
6. Cataract surgery	C75	92 622
7. Tonsillectomy	F34	74 751
8. Correction of glue ear	D15	68 038
9. Hernia repair	T20	61 721
10. Hysterectomy	Q07	59 607

operations in England in 1992–93 (Department of Health 1993b). The list avoids one or two groups of operations that are huge clusters of procedures and tries to list individual operation types. Two of the first three procedures are diagnostic. Endoscopies and cystoscopies alone account for almost 9% of all operations. Diagnostic procedures of all types (outside and inside the 10 selected procedures) account for over 15% of all operations in England. The second and fourth ranked procedures are two groups that are dominated by termination of pregnancy and the gynaecological procedure, dilatation and curettage. The complexity of the coding system means that some terminations of pregnancy occur in both Q10 and Q11 groupings but, nevertheless, these two procedures are amongst the most common undertaken in England.

Amongst these 10 common operations we find 5 procedures which are the subject of considerable disagreement amongst surgeons, regarding whether the operation should be used at all and, if so, on which patients and at what time.

1. Curettage of the uterus (rank 4), commonly called D&C, is a minor gynaecological operation that is used both diagnostically and as part of treatment. It is the fourth most common

operation in England, and English surgeons use the procedure at a rate per population which is 6 times higher than in the United States of America (Couter et al 1993). A leading article in the *British Medical Journal* (Lewis 1993) described the operation as 'diagnostically inaccurate and therapeutically useless'.

2. Ranked fifth is surgical removal of teeth, which usually means the removal of wisdom teeth. It is one of the most common operations performed in oral surgery, but this operation is also subject to considerable scepticism (Shepherd 1994). In the *British Medical Journal* it was argued that clinical audit suggests that rates of surgical intervention for the removal of wisdom teeth could be reduced and that more rational decision-making is needed. It argued that the cost:benefit ratio of this procedure is very poor and that little evidence exists of a link between levels of morbidity and undertaking the operation.

3. Ranked seventh on Table 3.1 is the removal of tonsils, described earlier as discretionary surgery.

4. Ranked ninth is the hysterectomy operation, which has for years been regarded as one of the operations most susceptible to surgical discretion with claims that at least one-third of all hysterectomies undertaken are unnecessary (Finkel 1988).

5. Ranked tenth is drainage of the middle ear. Glue ear was said to be one of the most popular reasons for elective surgery in children in England. A leader in the *British Medical Journal* in January 1993 described the growth in this operation as an epidemic (De Melker 1993). The article stated that GPs have a crucial role in reducing this surgical activity, by surveillance and reassuring parents of most affected children that the problems they have encountered would resolve themselves without any further action or adverse consequences. A letter responding to that article suggested that for once the poor might have a considerable advantage if they had to wait a long time for treatment: 'In Britain, waiting times for being seen in an out-patient clinic, followed by those for surgery, ensure that most children have waited a considerable time before grommet insertion, adenoidectomy, or a combination can be performed. This waiting time will in most cases select out those children whose effusions are short lived.'(Marshall & Narula 1993) At the time of the 1992 general election, the NHS was criticized for failing to have treated a young girl called Jennifer. Despite the fact that she had been waiting a

long time for an operation in the NHS, it may well have been that the best evaluated medical intervention and advice available was not to operate.

In fact, few of the operations listed in the top 10 can be classed as carrying a high degree of scientific approval. Only hernia repair and cataract surgery are widely regarded as sound surgical procedures, with a high degree of clinical agreement about which patients will benefit from the operation and at what point the operation should be done. It has to be said that even for these procedures there is disagreement about the point of intervention, but the operation itself is certainly seen to be a technical success. Repair of hernia is widely regarded as an effective operation, although there remain substantial variations in recurrence rate following the hernia repair (Williams et all 1994c). Cataract surgery is seen as a highly cost-effective intervention and is widely regarded as making a significant contribution to an improvement in the quality of life for many elderly people. In this case, the major problem seems to be agreeing the precise criteria which determine whether or not a cataract should be removed. Eight different criteria are widely used, and the most frequent criteria (that of determining visual acuity) shows that surgeons exercise widely differing views about when to operate (Williams et al 1994a). Patients who undergo eye tests might expect there to be some agreement about distance or size of letters that would indicate the need for an operation, but no such measures are universally accepted by surgeons. Even where large groups of surgeons agree criteria, the actual thresholds used for deciding whether to operate still vary considerably (Mordue et all 1994).

MAJOR OPERATIONS NOT IN THE TOP 10

The top 10 surgical procedures exclude some of the major operations that are well known to the public, such as heart surgery and joint replacement surgery. These operations are known to be effective, but the issue at stake is the point at which surgeons decide to intervene.

Coronary artery bypass surgery was said to have been inappropriate or equivocal in over 40% of the cases in the Trent Region (Gray et al 1990), and in a random selection of hospitals in the Western United States this proportion ranged from 23% to 63% (Winslow et al 1988). Brook pointed out that studies consistently find rates of care that are less than appropriate, at levels which are too high to be justified being ignored (Brook 1994). In total hip replacement surgery, the absence of universally agreed criteria upon which to determine the point of intervention leaves considerable doubt about how surgeons select which individual should undergo the operation (Williams et al 1994b). In the case of knee replacement surgery, we discover that there are some prostheses (replacement parts) that clearly do not work and should no longer be used when undertaking the operation (Williams et al 1994d). The failure rates following total knee replacements continue to show wide variation and there is concern at the continued use of certain TKR prostheses that have been discredited in the literature.

SHADES OF UNCERTAINTY

You do not need to have a medical degree to discover the great uncertainties and disagreements regarding surgical intervention. One of the great strengths of medicine is its willingness to discuss openly in medical and other journals its successes, failures and disagreements. What is perhaps surprising is the relatively low level of scientific evaluation of surgical and medical procedures. It has been estimated that less than 15% of health service intervention has been evaluated and proven to be beneficial (Hoare 1992).

Before a surgeon has even met his patient, a whole host of variables come into play: the thresholds of pain and discomfort that patients are prepared to put up with, the different opinions of the general practitioners who refer patients and the different levels of resources that are available for the surgeon to work with. The decision of a general practitioner as to whether or not to refer a patient for a second opinion can commonly show at least a three- or fourfold variation which cannot be explained by the characteristics of the patient, the geography of the practice or the case mix of those patients (Wilkin & Dornan 1990). The consultant negotiates the level or rate at which he sees out-patients by determining how many clinics he has during the week, how many patients he will see in each clinic and how many specialist referrals will be seen within those clinics or at additional specialist clinics.

Once patient and surgeon come face to face a range of decisions confront the surgeon. The choices are wide and over the years the following types of decision have been made. Some surgeons will select:

1. Operations which turn out to be ineffective or even harmful (Department of Health 1993a).
2. Operations that are largely needed for cosmetic reasons. This in no way suggests that the operation should not be undertaken, merely that it should be examined carefully in the light of competing calls from patients who need operations for life-threatening or debilitating conditions. No operation type can be classified as solely cosmetic, but nevertheless a substantial proportion of varicose vein and squint surgery, much plastic surgery and many general lump and bump removals are undertaken for cosmetic reasons only.
3. Operations on a basis that can only be described as fashion rather than clinical need. As the number of tonsil removals dropped there seemed to be a huge increase in the number of operations on patients with glue ear. Within a year of the introduction of the innovatory treatment of duodenal ulcer by drugs, surgical treatment of ulcers stopped. Surgeons then opted for other procedures, particularly gall bladder operations and now laparoscopy, which Bevan and Devlin (1994) suggest is a dubious use of resources.
4. Operations which are, in the main, highly effective, but for which the point of intervention cannot yet be scientifically determined. There is considerable scope for deciding at what point one removes a cataract or replaces a hip or knee.
5. Operations on patients selected by different priority criteria than those used by other colleagues. Some patients will be judged to be less in need of treatment than others, and will not be selected for surgery or even not seen by the surgeon. For an operation such as a coronary artery bypass graft, clinicians have developed very specific indications as to who might most appropriately undergo the operation, and yet it is found that many of those who do not meet the criteria undergo the operation (Grey et al 1990, Winslow et al 1988), and that many who do meet the criteria do not get the operation (London Implementation Group 1993).

It is commonly claimed that one of the causes of long waiting lists in Britain is the infinity of demand. It would appear that the need for surgery is not so much infinite as uncertain. The need for effective surgery cannot be infinite. We do not all need our hips and knees replaced and our wisdom teeth and gall bladders removed. It may be that the demand for surgical operations is greater than we can afford, but it certainly cannot be infinite. Given the claims about huge levels of unnecessary surgery, it would seem that we should try to ensure not that we do more operations overall, but that we reduce the number of inappropriate operations and replace them with operations that are appropriate. Politicians all too frequently claim how well the NHS is doing by citing an increase in the number of operations. If that increase is merely achieved by doing more inappropriate surgery, the NHS is not helping the nation's health or its finances.

PUTTING DISCRETION INTO CONTEXT

The purpose of this chapter has not been to criticize the lack of scientific knowledge, the lack of consensus over existing knowledge, or the inadequacies of the scientific approach of medicine over the past century. We have genuine and serious gaps in our scientific knowledge but, in the main, the scientific and medical community is consistently trying to bridge these gaps. What needs to be acknowledged is that there remains a large amount of discretion that each surgeon can, and does, exercise. The range is so large that it affects the total amount of surgery that is undertaken and also who receives and who does not receive surgical intervention. These problems are seriously compounded by the level of resources that are available – a subject that has not even been touched on in this chapter. Clearly, each surgeon has to operate within the constraints of the facilities available to him and these, too, affect his clinical decision-making. This chapter has not set out to claim or prove that any financial considerations (the ability to earn money from private practice) actually determines decisions or choices. It merely points out that the range of clinical discretion is so wide that it would be possible for some clinicians to take this factor into account in the decision-making process. This does not amount to evidence that there is any consistent patterning of the way in which decisions are made for the benefit of any groups of patients, be it on the grounds of age, colour, ability to pay or any other basis.

Recently, I have had two particularly lengthy debates with surgeon friends about the ethics of private practice that have helped me realize just how much strain our society places on consultant colleagues by allowing them to work in both the private sector and the NHS. One admitted to me that the pressures are so different that his inclination when faced with an NHS patient is to seek conservative forms of treatment and resort to surgery only after having considered all other alternatives. When faced by a private patient his first reaction is to operate, in order to show something is being done. He suspects that the two cultures encourage him to react differently when faced by the same category of patient. My other friend took the opposite view and argued that he operates more readily in the NHS than in the private sector. They are both highly regarded and competent surgeons and I would happily be referred to either, should the need arise. What I do know is that neither has sufficient scientific support to make consistent decisions. If these two men, who undertake very little private practice, find so much scope to vary their decisions about whether and when they operate, how easy it must be for other surgeons to alter the balance of their work between the private sector and the NHS, for reasons other than the clinical need of the patient.

A tale of two cities?

Both cities are served by surgeons who have wide discretion in deciding whether and when patients need to be operated on. It is uncertain whether the different health care systems lead to the surgeons making different decisions in each city. They have the scope to do so, but no one has the data to know whether it happens or not.

Consultants' workload in the NHS

This chapter sets out to discover how much operating consultants do in the NHS. We need this information for two reasons. First, what do we get in return for a £40 000 per year salary and, secondly, are surgeons operating safely? Surgeons tell us that if they do not operate frequently enough they lose their skills (Devlin 1994) and that would mean paying them to do little work and for some of it to be unsafe. On the other hand, if we force them to do too much work, that might also lead to unsafe operating and, once again, we would not be getting value for money. The problem for those of us who are not medically qualified is that we are not sure what is too few or too many, nor do we know what the right level should be.

There are just over 20 000 consultants in the United Kingdom, most of whom specialize in various types of medical and diagnostic work (Monopolies and Mergers Commission 1994b). Only 5145 are consultant surgeons and a further 2754 are consultant anaesthetists. British surgeons have a longer training than most other professions in the UK and a longer training than surgeons in other countries. From the time a medical student first goes to university it will be at least 12 and it could be 20 years before he or she is appointed as a consultant surgeon. That period will include many years in training as a junior doctor under the supervision of senior surgeons, as well as extensive and difficult courses and examinations. In Britain, virtually all surgeons take up their first appointment in the NHS. It is not compulsory to do so, but an immediate career in private practice has, to date, been most unlikely as few private insurance companies will recognize a consultant unless he holds an NHS appointment.

All surgeons receive the same basic training, but later specialize in treating specific parts of the human body. The main groups of surgeons in England and Wales are shown in Table 4.1 (Allen 1993). Each branch of surgery has its own balance of workload and its own needs for resources. The balance between the amount of time required assessing patients in clinics compared with the time spent operating on patients varies enormously between specialties. Cardiac surgeons, for instance, spend relatively little time on out-patient work (because much of this is undertaken by consultant cardiologists) and require more operating theatre time because of the length of time needed for the complicated major heart surgery they perform. Ophthalmologists,

Table 4.1 Number of consultant surgeons in the main surgical specialities – England and Wales 1992

Name of specialty	Main focus of surgery	Number
General surgery	Abdomen/gall bladder	1054
Gynaecology (including Obstetrics)	Female reproductive organs	880
Orthopaedics	Bones and joints	832
Ophthalmology	Eyes	495
Otorhinolaryngology	Ear, nose and throat	429
Oral surgery	Teeth and gums	261
Urology	Urinary/genital organs and kidneys	245
Cardio-thoracic	Heart and chest	143
Plastic surgery	Reconstruction	134
Neuro-surgery	Brain	103
Paediatric surgery	Children	50
Total		4626
Anaesthetists		2342

Source:
Medical and dental staffing prospectus in the NHS in England and Wales 1992.
Health Trends Vol 25 No 4 1993

on the other hand, can spend over half their time in out-patient and day care settings and use only a couple of operating theatre sessions per week. The differing needs of the specialties for operating lists, and the variations in the types of operations performed, even in the same specialty, means that it is difficult to talk about the work done by an 'average' surgeon.

Any attempt to measure the workload of surgeons needs to take account of, at least, five factors.

1. Surgeons have a wide range of tasks, other than the purely technical function of operating. Much of their work has qualitative aspects which are extremely difficult and sometimes impossible to measure.
2. Measuring operative workload is difficult, because much of the data required is difficult to get hold of and some of the data which is available is inaccurate.
3. Operative workload varies enormously between specialties and between surgeons in the same specialties. There are huge differences between the proportions of emergency and planned surgery and in the complexity of operations. Some take only 5 minutes and others can last 7–8 hours or even longer. Any attempt to measure a surgeon's operative workload has to take account of these case mix variations.
4. Surgeons can be constrained by the level of physical resources provided. We cannot attempt to measure surgical activity without taking account of the number of theatre facilities, hospital beds and other resources that are required to back up each surgeon.
5. Consultants have a variable level of support from junior surgical staff. Not only do teams vary in size, but the level of competence and seniority of junior staff differs between surgical teams and over time. The amount of support given to the consultant by juniors and the amount of support and training the consultant needs to give to juniors can vary enormously.

THE IMMEASURABLE PROFESSION

One of the most frequent observations made about surgeons is that they 'love to operate'. All other elements of a surgeon's activity are seen as preparatory or consequential to their fundamental role – operating. The surgeon's working week involves a range of activities associated with conducting an operation. These include attendance at out-patient clinics and ward rounds, teaching junior staff, conducting research, undertaking audit and fulfilling many administrative but vital functions, such as writing patients' discharge letters to GPs. To some extent, therefore, examining consultants' workload by concentrating on the amount of surgery undertaken is simplistic. It could be argued that the consultant's role in the NHS is that of a team leader and that they are primarily there to ensure that operations are performed, but not necessarily by themselves. One surgeon told me that the most important thing he did was not to operate, but to make the decision of whether or not to operate.

The notion that consultant surgeons should mainly be decision-making team leaders can, however, be overstated. We do not spend 12–20 years training someone simply to train others. Surgeons are trained to operate and that is what we expect them to do. Most patients would prefer to be operated on by a highly trained and competent surgeon and the NHS and the medical profession itself are both committed to having a higher proportion of consultants, in order that more patients can benefit from such skills. Nor is the 'team leader' argument applied in the private sector, where it is assumed that virtually all operating will be conducted by the qualified consultant.

Patients expect surgeons to spend most of their week operating, because they understand that is what they have been trained to do. Surgeons are expected to keep up to date in technical terms and operate on a sufficiently large number of patients to maintain their skills at a high level. It was Florence Nightingale who first noted significant differences between the success rates of surgical units operating on soldiers in the Crimean War. In more recent years, surgical literature (e.g. Luft et al 1979, Luft et al 1990, Hannan et al 1991) has looked at the relationship between the volume of surgery undertaken and the results obtained. A simplistic theme running through this literature is that 'practice makes perfect'. As one of Britain's leading surgeons, and champion of the need for improved clinical audit, pointed out, 'There is a well known relationship between the volume of surgery a surgeon does and his outcome ... A surgeon needs to keep his hand in ...' (Devlin 1994). The more of one type of operation surgeons do, the better they become at it. The low volume operators are often seen as less skilful and, sometimes, even dangerous. But the moment the press and government start advocating the publication of league tables for surgeons which show variable death rates (Laurance 1993) there is an immediate defensive outcry protesting that the workload of surgeons cannot be fairly measured (e.g. Anon. 1993).

POOR QUALITY DATA

Even if we are prepared to ignore the pleas to refrain from measuring the workload of surgeons, we soon encounter practical difficulties. If we accept that operating is an important part of a surgeon's workload, how do we then go about examining the number of operations a surgeon does? The NHS cannot answer the simple question, 'How many operations does a surgeon do in a week?' The data is simply not available. The NHS regularly counts how many operations are done, it even records what types of operation are done, but it does not collect routine information about *who* performs them. The data is written down – but not in a place where anyone can use it. The casenotes of each patient and the theatre register have for years been the only documents which record the name of the actual surgeon who undertakes the operation. The most detailed information appears in each patient's casenotes, but these do not tell us how many operations were done in a particular theatre on any particular day. Casenotes are filed in a sequence that allows staff to retrieve the notes (usually casenote number linked to an alphabetical index) and are not in a date order by operation.

The best method of obtaining information about theatre activity has usually been to study the theatre register. My experience of examining hundreds of theatre registers has revealed many difficulties. For decades, theatre registers have consisted of large, old-fashioned ledgers, in which theatre sisters, nurses and surgeons enter the name of each patient operated on. The register usually includes details of drugs administered, swab counts and other basic details about the patient and the operation. In most cases the name of the operating surgeon and assistant are recorded, together with the anaesthetist.

The trouble with this system of recording is that it does not tell you whether or not the consultant surgeon was present. If listed as the operating surgeon or assistant, it is reasonable to assume that the consultant was there for at least some of the operating session, but the absence of a name does not necessarily mean that the consultant was not present. He or she may have actually been in the theatre observing and training the junior, or close at hand in the theatre suite available to be called at a second's notice, but the name is not necessarily logged in the register. No theatre register could distinguish between either of those modes, or tell us if the consultant was actually on the golf course. Theatre registers are not easily analysed and require hours of careful work before any patterns of activity can be ascertained. For this reason, few managers have the faintest idea what their surgeons do. It is only in recent years, with the advent of computerized theatre systems, that any form of analysis has become easier. But these systems are not universally installed, and where they are in use, different and incompatible systems are available. Moreover, some are not yet trusted by surgeons or managers to produce reliable information.

STANDARDIZING FOR CASE MIX

Even if we could ascertain how many operations each surgeon does, the information would carry little weight with surgeons themselves because their workload has not been 'standardized'. Operations can take anything from a few minutes to many hours. To convert the numbers of operations performed into actual time spent operating, it is necessary to record the start and finish time of each operation. One immediately encounters two difficulties. First, what is the precise start time of an operation – when the patient is wheeled into the theatre suite – when the anaesthetist starts to give an anaesthetic – when the surgeon first puts knife to skin? There are similarly 'different' finishing times and some of these might overlap as one patient might still be on the theatre table when the next is already under an anaesthetic. So, recording the length of the operation is not a simple process and not all hospitals would agree about which times to use. The second, more fundamental problem is that the vast majority of theatre registers simply do not record any start and finish times. If it is not recorded, theatre registers cannot be used to find out how long the operations actually took.

In the absence of the more recently introduced computerized recording systems, the study of theatre usage has had to rely on various forms of classification produced by surgeons. These classification systems group operations into categories according to the estimated length of operating time involved. One such system has been developed by BUPA (The British United Provident Association Ltd. 1993), who have classified hundreds of operations as either minor, intermediate, major, major plus or complex major. Each group represents an increasing amount of required operating time and thus surgeons' fees in the private sector correspondingly climb from minor up through the scale to complex major. The scale of operating times is based on the calculation that intermediate operations take about 1 hour. The other classifications are scaled to the equivalent of an intermediate operation as shown in Table 4.2.

The estimated times needed have been based on studies of actual times taken, but only represent a set of averages and clearly there can be great differences between times taken within each group. One deficiency of the system is that the minimum average time quoted is half an hour and many surgical procedures take only a few minutes. However, whilst managers, surgeons and researchers can find imperfections in this method, it does have a wide level of acceptance. Using the system illustrates how standardizing simple counts of numbers can produce differing estimates of time spent (Table 4.3). The relationship between the number of operations and the time taken varies between specialties and within specialties, but it is fair to say that the average operation in Britain is calculated as lasting between 1 hour and 1 hour 15 minutes.

Table 4.2   Converting operation numbers to operating time

Type of operation	Intermediate equivalent	Estimated time needed hours	minutes
Minor	0. 5	0	30
Intermediate	1.0	1	00
Major	1.75	1	45
Major plus	2.2	2	12
Complex major	4.0	4	00

Source:
The British United Provident Association Ltd, 1993 Working with BUPA: a guide for specialists, Section 1, Schedule of procedures

Table 4.3 The relationship between the number of operations and operating time

Number of operations	Estimate of hours spent	Average time per operation		Study
		hours	minutes	
4374	6282	1	26	Bath orthopaedic (Pozo & Jones 1993)
5487	6177	1	08	BUPA Norwich (Laing 1992a)
4865	5605	1	09	General surgery in Somerset 1994 (O'Leary & Collins 1994)
57 308	51 024	0	53	ENT in Trent Region 1983–85 (George & Braxier 1991)

CONSTRAINED BY RESOURCES?

It should be self-evident that the more operating lists per week surgeons are given, the more operations they do. Data presented later in this chapter and elsewhere in the book will show that general surgery and urology surgeons, with 3 or 4 lists per week, usually do more operations than ophthalmologists who only have around 2 lists per week. Similarly, within specialties, surgeons with 3 or 4 lists per week usually do more than those with only 1 or 2 lists per week.

Surgeons are not in control of their own destinies in the NHS. The number of operations they are able to undertake is invariably constrained by a lack of resources. In my experience, newly appointed surgeons are generally very difficult to please in this respect because they want to operate more frequently than the system can allow. In an early draft of this book I commented on ENT surgeons having 3 operating sessions each week. An ENT surgeon who read my draft commented 'I have spent my consultant life of over 20 years with only 2 lists per week.' He was willing to do more operating but had never been given sufficient resources to do so (personal communication 1994a).

The level of theatre sessions provided per surgeon is not standard across the country. There are College guidelines which recommend the number of lists that surgeons think they should be provided with (e.g. British Association of Otolaryngologists

1986, British Medical Association Orthopaedic Subcommittee (undated), The Royal College of Surgeons of England 1990, College of Ophthalmologists 1988) but individual health authorities and hospitals do not always provide the number recommended. Sometimes this is because there are not enough theatres, sometimes a theatre is available but there is insufficient cash to staff it and sometimes there are not enough beds or other facilities to support the operating theatre sessions. These problems often have a long history, and there are highly variable levels of provision, town by town across the country.

More recently, the financial pressures felt by some hospitals towards the end of the financial year, or as a result of rationalization of resources, have led to reduction and loss of theatre sessions. In an 8-month period in 1993 the Royal College of Surgeons reported (Beecham 1994a) that 44% of surgical divisions had been told to stop or reduce some activity. The amount of work that a surgeon can do in a week is not simply dependent on the individual's inclination and ability.

THE CONTRIBUTION OF THE JUNIOR SURGEON

In the absence of routine data systems regarding who performs operations, I was forced to turn to individual studies of theatre records to try and find out which surgeon undertakes which operation. Over the past few years I have led a team responsible for studying some of Britain's worst waiting list problems. These studies have given us access to over 200 groups of surgeons spread over half of the nation's health authorities. In over 50 of these studies it was necessary to undertake a detailed examination of theatre registers. In this process we recorded not only the operation undertaken, but which surgeon was listed as undertaking the operation. Theatre registers sometimes record that more than one surgeon is involved in an operation. Where that was the case we always credited the consultant surgeon with the operation and assumed they were present and assisting. Where the consultant's name did not appear in the theatre register, we did not take this to imply that the consultant was not present, but noted that the consultant was not recorded as undertaking the operation nor listed as an assistant at that operation. Such operations were credited to the junior.

In over 36 000 operations studied, the consultant was recorded as undertaking or assisting at less than half. Table 4.4 and Figure 4.1 show the variations between specialties with juniors undertaking only 32% of major coronary artery by-pass surgery, but doing 70% of ENT surgery. There are also wide variations between the hospital sites studied which serves to emphasize how difficult it is to talk about 'average' or typical surgical practice in Britain. In ophthalmology the huge range in the number of operations done by juniors – from 3% to 64% – is explained by the differing staffing levels in different types of hospital. The 3% figure was from a district general hospital with minimal junior staff cover, whilst the 64% figure was from a teaching hospital with a large number of juniors.

The ENT figures were somewhat surprising and revealed a very high proportion of work undertaken by junior staff in a number of hospitals with severe waiting list problems. It is thought that these hospitals were probably not typical of district general hospitals in Britain and we would not expect the proportion of work done by juniors in ENT to be quite as high as shown in this study. Although the orthopaedic studies are probably

Table 4.4 Split of operations between consultants and juniors

Specialty	Dates	Number of studies	Number of cases	Operated on by consultant	Operated on by juniors	% done by juniors	% range among studies
Trauma and ortho-paedics	1986–93	22	16 529	7090	9439	57	32–86
Opthal-mology	1987–92	8	5256	2807	2449	47	3–64
General surgery	1986–91	4	3340	1698	1642	49	27–59
Urology	1993	1	1501	465	1036	69	
ENT	1986–91	8	4980	1474	3506	70	67–93
Plastic surgery	1989–90	4	2688	915	1773	66	58–70
CABG	1993	9	1353	915	438	32	14–48
Gynae-cology	1988	1	491	320	171	35	
Totals	1986–93	57	36 138	15 684	20 454	57	3–93

Source:
57 studies by Inter-Authority Comparisons and Consultancy (University of Birmingham) between 1986 and 1993

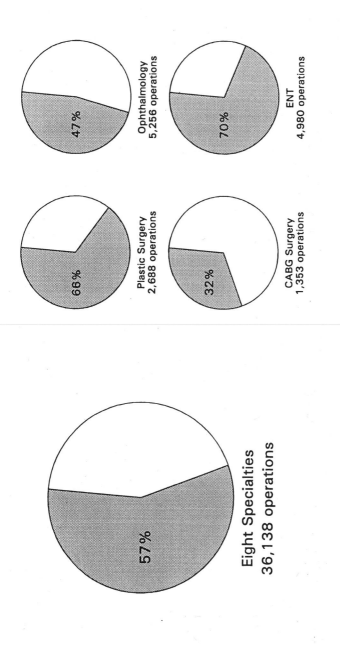

Figure 4.1 Percentage of operations undertaken by junior surgeons

Source:
57 theatre studies 1986–93

more representative of British surgical practice, it should be noted that they included a number of major centres in which the proportion of emergency surgery was somewhat lower than the average district general hospital. Given that emergency operations are more frequently done by juniors than by consultants, it might be that in this specialty the proportion of work done by juniors is slightly higher than that shown in the study.

From the evidence available it seems reasonable to conclude that out of any 100 operations performed in Britain at least 50–55 will be undertaken by juniors. This does not necessarily indicate that consultants were absent from the operating theatre. However, a Royal College of Surgeons' study (Campling et al 1993) of 826 patients who had died following an operation by a junior surgeon, showed that consultants were not present for over 60% of those operations. This study, and other observations of surgical practice, suggest that it is likely that the majority of the operations undertaken by juniors are performed without a consultant present.

MEASURING THE IMMEASURABLE
The average surgeon

The workload of individual surgeons is not recorded at hospital, health authority or Department of Health level. Data is, however, gathered on a specialty basis, which means that we can get some idea of the surgical activity of teams (i.e. the consultant and their juniors) within specialties. Given that we know the number of operations performed, the number of operating sessions held and the number of consultants in each specialty, we can calculate the average operative workload per team. Table 4.5 shows the average workload in England in 1991–92 for four different specialties. It shows how different specialties perform in terms of the number of patients they operate on in a year and also shows the average weekly availability of operating sessions. The fact that general surgical teams do twice as many operations as ophthalmology teams is likely to be influenced by the number of theatre sessions available, but as discussed earlier, other factors influence surgical throughput. For example, the fact that ENT surgeons do more operations per year in less theatre sessions than orthopaedic surgeons is likely to be due to the higher proportion of minor and intermediate cases in ENT.

Table 4.5 Operative workload in four specialities England 1991–92

Specialty	Operations per team per year	Average weekly theatre sessions per consultant
Ophthalmology	508	2.6
Trauma and orthopaedics	775	4.1
Ear Nose and Throat	834	3.5
General surgery and urology	1046	4.8

Source:
Calculated from base data about number of theatre sessions and number of operations obtained from Department of Health returns KH08 1991/1992
Consultant data came from Medical Manpower Census DC20 1990/1991

An examination of the workload of teams on a district by district basis across the country shows that the averages per specialty in Table 4.5 mask wide variations. There is usually more than a threefold difference between the district with the lowest numbers of operations per year and those with the highest numbers. In ophthalmology, for instance, although the average was 508 operations per team per year, there were teams doing less than 100 operations per year whilst others did over 1500. Figure 4.2 shows these wide variations. Surgeons and managers offer various explanations for these large differences and commonly cite the variations in case mix and level of resources as the two principle factors.

On the basis of the study of the workload of junior surgeons described earlier, we can re-examine the earlier data on the workload of the average surgical team. Table 4.6 shows the number of operations conducted per year by the average consultant and his team of juniors (first column). If we assume that half of the operations are undertaken by juniors and then divide the annual figure by 46 weeks (to allow 6 weeks for holidays) we can see that the average surgeon does between 6 and 11 operations per week, depending on the specialty involved. If sick leave and study leave were added into the calculation the average workload would be slightly higher. In the main it is the consultant, rather than the junior, who does the more complicated surgery. The average personal weekly operating volume of 6–11 operations

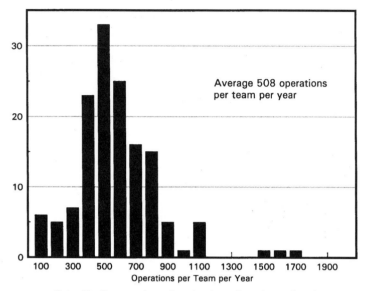

Note: The figures underneath each column show the number of
operations performed up to 100, 200, 300, etc.

Figure 4.2 Annual number of operations per surgical team per district in
ophthalmology – England

Source:
IACC Time Series Indicators 1991–92

Table 4.6 Estimated number of operations per consultant per week

Speciality	Recorded number of operations per team per year	Estimated number of operations per consultant per week
Ophthalmology	508	6
Trauma and orthopaedics	775	8
Ear nose and throat	834	9
General surgery and urology	1046	11

Source:
Calculated from base data about number of theatre sessions and number of
operations obtained from Department of Health returns KH08 1991/1992
Consultant data came from Medical Manpower Census DC20 1990/1991

Table 4.7   Problems with estimating workload of consultant surgeons

Assumptions	Facts
50% of operating done by junior	The actual proportion ranges (at least) from 3% to 93%
All surgeons perform at the same rate as the average team in their district	We know there are huge variations amongst teams within districts
Assessments of time based on BUPA scale are reliable	The actual time of operation can be less than or greater than the average time given

then has to be multiplied by the case mix factor, which might be somewhere between 53 minutes and 1 hour 26 minutes per operation (Table 4.3). On that assumption it could be estimated that most consultants do between 5 and 15 hours operating per week.

The calculated averages mask a high degree of variation and are based on a number of assumptions that are not always valid (Table 4.7). This means that some surgeons may spend less than 5 hours per week operating in the NHS and others will spend more than 15 hours.

A 5% sample of British consultant surgeons

Mathematical averages, ranges and calculations do not provide a detailed or adequate description of what consultant surgeons do. Over the past 5 years my team from Birmingham University were invited to work on waiting list problems in over 100 British health authorities. This work gave us the opportunity to meet nearly 1000 consultants and to gain access to data about their workload. In the process of investigating the causes of long waiting lists, the team studied the provision and use of resources, particularly in relation to beds, surgeons, out-patient clinics and theatre sessions. On many occasions this necessitated a detailed study of theatre activity and, as a result, we are able to present data about the operative workload of 274 consultant surgeons-more than 5% of all British surgeons.

The studies were always conducted over a period of at least 13 weeks and in each case surgeons and theatre staff were asked to identify what they considered to be typical periods (i.e. we

avoided major holiday breaks and closures of theatre for mainte-
nance). The study periods extended over 5 years and thus do not
represent an atypical time in the life of the NHS. Data collection
and analysis was made directly from the original or photocopied
theatre registers by a team of six staff well used to data collection
and analysis. Most had worked for long periods of time in the
NHS, but none were medically qualified. Data transcription
errors are likely to be relatively small, but the coding of operations may have been a little less reliable for unusual and less
frequent operations (although in each specialty we used a clinical advisor to help with any coding difficulties).

The most likely source of systematic error was the original
recording of the name of the operating surgeon. We had to
accept the accuracy and descriptions in the theatre registers
themselves. In all cases the presence or absence of a surgeon
cannot be absolutely guaranteed by the presence or absence of
his or her name in the theatre register. The study obviously had
its imperfections, but we used a consistent method over the 5
years. The results of each individual study were presented to
representatives of the surgeons and managers concerned in
each hospital and the methods used and the results obtained
were never seriously challenged. I believe that the study
provides a reasonably accurate account of operations undertaken.

I have displayed the actual number of operations per week
over a 3-month period, by adding all the operations undertaken
by each consultant and dividing by the number of weeks. Whilst
major holiday periods were always avoided, it could be argued
that at least 8 weeks of every year are not available to a surgeon
because of holidays and study leave and thus about 15% of each
period is likely to see consultant absence. This would mean a 13-
week period might only include 11 working weeks. A surgeon
doing 4.7 operations per week over a 13-week period would
actually be doing 5.4 operations per week in the available 11
working weeks during that period. Such a re-calculation is
marginal.

In each case a minimum of 13 weeks was analysed and, for
192 of the consultants we studied, every operating theatre
session they undertook during that time. For the remaining 83
surgeons, the work undertaken at their main hospital base was
studied, but some sessions undertaken in other NHS hospitals

Table 4.8   Number of operations per week for 274 surgeons

Specialty	No. of surgeons	Average no. per week	Range	No. with 3 or fewer cases/week
Trauma and orthopaedics	120	4.6	1–10	25
Ophthalmology	48	4.4	1–10	11
Cardiac surgery	39	4.3	2–11	6
ENT surgery	30	3.2	1–9	16
General surgery and urology	19	7.2	3–12	1
Plastic surgery	14	6.1	3–12	1
Gynaecology	4	6.2	6–8	0
Total	274	4.7	1–12	60

Source:
Studies by IACC between 1986 and 1993

were not. Where this was the case the workload at the main hospital was adjusted pro-rata. If a surgeon had 2 lists per week at the main hospital and 1 per week in another hospital, the workload of the 2 sessions was increased by 50% to calculate the average weekly workload. This would sometimes have the effect of under-estimating the consultant's workload and on other occasions, producing an over-estimate. In both groups the resultant workload figures were very similar, suggesting that the method of estimating was not over- or undergenerous.

The results of these studies showed that this group of 274 British surgeons averaged 4.7 operations per week. None exceeded an average of 12 cases per week, and 20% of them did 3 or fewer cases per week. (Table 4.8, Fig. 4.3) The patterns of activity varied between specialties.

Trauma and orthopaedic surgery

The largest group studied was a sample of 120 trauma and orthopaedic surgeons. In the main, consultants concentrated on planned operations and the vast bulk of emergency operations were undertaken by junior staff. These 120 consultants operated on between 1 and 10 patients per week and the majority (60%) undertook 4, 5 or 6 operations per week (Fig. 4.4). A fifth of the surgeons operated on 3 or fewer patients per week and, at the

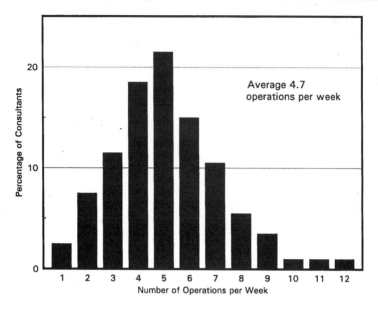

Figure 4.3 Weekly operative workload of 274 consultant surgeons

Source:
57 theatre studies 1986–93

other end of the scale, a fifth of the consultants did 7 or more operations per week.

There was no discernible difference between the group of 74 surgeons for whom we had complete data and the 46 surgeons for whom data was only partially collected. The first group averaged 4.5 operations per week, the latter group averaged 4.7 operations per week, and the whole group produced a figure of 4.6 operations per week.

Ophthalmology

In ophthalmology most operations were planned surgery with only a very small proportion of emergency work. In this specialty, again, there was a wide range of workload, from 1 to 10 operations per week. The majority (62%) of consultants performed 4, 5 or 6 operations per week, and as in orthopaedics about 20% of surgeons did 3 or fewer operations per week (Fig. 4.5). Of the 48 surgeons studied, for 37 of them we had full data for all work undertaken. For the 11 where only lists at the main

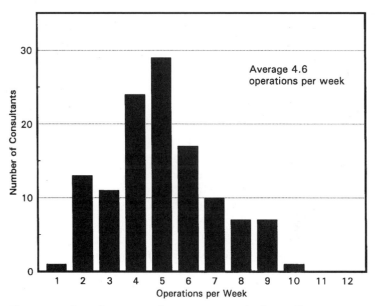

Figure 4.4   Operations per week – 120 trauma and orthopaedic surgeons

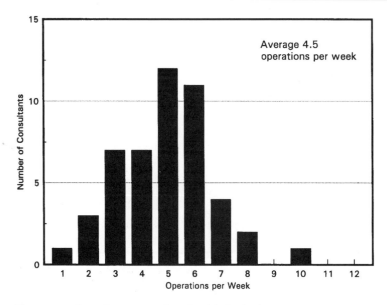

Figure 4.5   Operations per week – 48 ophthalmologists

Source Figures 4.4, 4.5:
Orthopaedic and Ophthalmology theatre studies 1986–93

hospital were studied the average workload seemed to be lower and it may be that our assumptions about the remaining lists were imperfect (i.e. perhaps they did more operations per week in units other than their main hospital).

Cardiac surgery

Unlike our studies of other specialties, the examination of cardiac surgery workload was not done as a result of studying in-patient waiting lists. The study of cardiac surgery was commissioned as part of a wider review of services in London and we were specifically requested to look at the workload of 39 consultant surgeons. Of these, 1 surgeon averaged 11 operations per week, but the remainder ranged from 2 to 7 operations per week, with an overall average of 4.3. In this specialty, 70% of surgeons undertook 4, 5 or 6 operations per week, with 15% undertaking 3 or fewer and 15% undertaking 7 or more (Fig. 4.6). In the case of cardiac surgery, it should be noted that these figures tend to overestimate the consultant workload. For 7 surgeons we were unable to separate out all of the work of the junior surgeons, which is why these 7 usually had a higher than average workload.

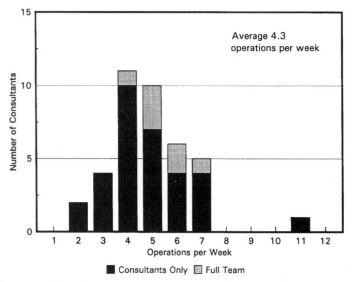

Figure 4.6 Operations per week – 39 cardiac surgeons

Source:
Cardiac surgery theatre studies 1992

One of the surprising findings of this study was that the academic units (with consultants who devoted a substantial proportion of their time to teaching and research commitment) averaged 5.4 cases per week, whilst the 25 NHS consultants, with less teaching and research commitment, only averaged 3.9 cases per week.

ENT surgery

In ENT only 30 surgeons were studied, and only just over half of those for their full weekly workload. The ENT sample produced remarkable results, with more than half of the surgeons doing 3 or fewer operations per week (Fig. 4.7). The surgeon who undertook the highest workload of 9 cases per week was actually a locum ENT surgeon who did not have his FRCS qualification (he did more minor surgery). The remaining 29 surgeons studied all did fewer than 7 operations per week, even though most of them had at least 3 operating sessions available to them. Most observers would regard these figures as unusually low and certainly not typical of ENT surgical activity.

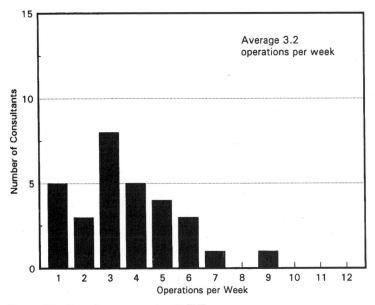

Figure 4.7   Operations per week – 30 ENT surgeons

Source:
ENT theatre studies 1986–93

Other specialties

Our studies covered 37 additional consultants in four other specialties and Figure 4.8 shows the weekly activity of this disparate group. Half of the surgeons undertook 6, 7 or 8 operations per week, with roughly one-quarter of the group doing 5 or fewer, and a further quarter doing 9 or more operations per week.

The results of the 5% sample of consultant activity give an average of just under 5 operations per week per surgeon. For individual specialties the averages ranged from a low of 3 to a high of 7 operations per week and for individual consultants the range was between 1 and 12 operations per week.

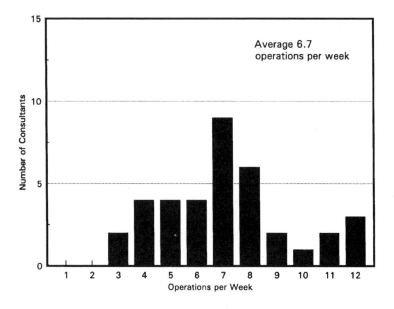

Figure 4.8 Operations per week – 37 consultants in four specialties (general surgery, plastic surgery, urology, gynaecology)

Source:
Theatre studies 1986–93

CAN THE VERY LOW FIGURES BE BELIEVED?

Our experience of using this type of analysis and our studies of actual theatre session start and finish times have consistently shown us that consultants tend to handle more major cases than junior surgeons, but the wide variations in numbers of operations per consultant is not explained by standardizing for time. We do not find that the surgeons with low numbers of operations are all doing highly complex and time-consuming surgery, neither are the high volume operators all doing minor and intermediate operations. One might have expected cardiac surgeons, who undertake valve replacement and heart and lung transplant surgery, to do far fewer operations than an ophthalmologist in a general hospital who mainly treats cataracts and squints. This study, however, finds a cardiac surgeon doing 10 major operations per week, whilst there are some ophthalmologists and many ENT surgeons doing 3 or fewer operations per week.

We re-examined the work of all 60 surgeons who did 3 or fewer operations per week and only in a small number of instances did we find that there was a complicated case mix which explained the low volume. There were 2 orthopaedic surgeons who did undertake very complex surgery and 5 professors whose teaching and research commitments might explain low operating volume. It might also be argued that the low volume of work undertaken by 6 cardiac surgeons is due to the specialty being dominated by complex major operations. But why do many of their colleagues operate on twice as many cases per week? The vast majority of low-volume operators did not undertake unusual, complex or time-consuming surgery. They were to be found in ordinary district general hospitals and teaching hospitals throughout Britain.

To illustrate this, the apparently low workloads of two ENT surgeons were independently assessed. The low-workload surgeons worked in the same industrial conurbation in England and in a 13-week period one surgeon personally conducted 11 operations and the other just 7. Neither had been on study leave, annual leave or sick leave for any substantial part of that period. I had thought that perhaps the surgeons specialized in extremely complex and lengthy operations, or that they may have had extremely onerous research and teaching commitments.

In order to cross check the first supposition I sent a list of the operations undertaken by each of the surgeons during the 13-week period to the two independent assessors. I listed the operations that had appeared in the theatre registers and asked each of the two assessors (who were consultant ENT surgeons) whether there was anything unusual about the operations, in terms of their complexity. I also asked for estimates of the amount of time it would take to undertake the two groups of 11 and 7 operations. In neither case did I tell the assessor over what period the work had been undertaken. Both assessors responded by saying there was nothing unusual about the case mix, and in the case of the 11 operations the work should have taken about 9 hours 30 minutes and the seven operations about 4 hours. In both cases the independent assessors had assumed that I was talking about 1 week's work for an ENT surgeon, when actually I had sent them the work of 13 weeks. In neither of the cases can it be claimed that the surgeons involved have extremely onerous teaching and research responsibilities.

Similar examinations revealed there were many surgeons among the group of 60 (doing 3 or fewer operations per week) whose level of operating could not be explained by the need to standardize the case mix. There had to be other reasons for the very low volume of surgery. Even if this set of surgeons are not typical of British surgical practice, they do illustrate that a minority are, for whatever reasons, unable or unwilling to do much operating in the NHS. To identify, almost by chance, a group of 60 consultant surgeons who do 3 or fewer NHS operations per week ought to raise questions about whether the NHS is making best use of an extremely valuable resource.

ARE THE 274 SURGEONS TYPICAL OF BRITISH PRACTICE?

This sample had two obvious biases. First, the group of surgeons was not representative of all specialties; some were not included at all and some were very over-represented (e.g. trauma and orthopaedics). The results, therefore, are not typical of all surgeons, but could be considered as representative of most of the specialties included. The second bias was that the vast majority of the surgeons studied worked in hospitals that had severe waiting list problems. The detailed studies of theatre registers were made because it was felt that either the allocation of sessions or the volume of work in sessions might have made some contribution to the waiting list problems. However, it is not easy to anticipate what sort of potential bias is given to the sample by the fact that the group of surgeons studied had particularly long waiting lists. Would we expect these surgeons to be working much harder than average in order to try and reduce these lists, or might we expect a low-volume workload to be contributing to the long waiting list? Rather than argue about how typical the sample is, perhaps it would be easier to compare how the sample performs against, first, the expectations of surgeons themselves; secondly, against the nationally available data described earlier in this chapter; and thirdly, against a similar study recently undertaken by an independent audit group.

Comparing the sample with surgeons' opinions

In 1989 I attended the annual scientific meeting of the Association of Professors of Orthopaedic Surgery, open to all orthopaedic consultants. I circulated a questionnaire to 161 consultants, professors and senior lecturers in orthopaedics. One of the questions asked was 'How many operations would you expect a consultant to perform in a week?' I received 76 replies to the question, and the answers ranged from 1 to 23. This group of consultants, who were biased towards academic and teaching units, expected consultants to be operating on an average of 8.4 patients per week. The figure is significantly higher than the actual number of 4.6 for the 120 orthopaedic surgeons studied, but it is interesting to note that a substantial proportion of the ranges overlap (Fig. 4.9). Only a minority of orthopaedic surgeons expected to operate on more than 10 cases per week, which is not far removed from the reality in the sample studied.

Comparing the sample with national statistics

An alternative way of assessing how typical this sample of surgeons might be, is to compare the workload with the aggregated figures examined earlier. At the beginning of this chapter, I described the annual number of operations per surgical team in England for the year 1991–92 (Fig. 4.2, Table 4.6). If we assume for a moment that half of the work was done by juniors and then further divide the workload by 46, we can create diagrams that

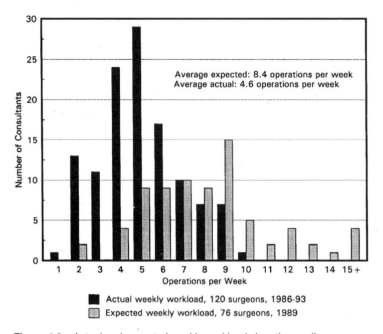

Figure 4.9 Actual and expected weekly workloads in orthopaedics

Source:
IACC theatre studies 1986–93, Survey of orthopaedic surgeons 1989

give a rough idea of how many operations are performed per consultant surgeon per week. Those figures can then be compared with the actual weekly workload of the surgeons in each specialty. This might enable us to make some assessment as to how typical that sample of 274 surgeons was compared with the rest of England.

In the case of ophthalmology the average workload was estimated at 5.5 cases per week and the actual figures recorded were closer to 4.5 per week. In Figure 4.10 the two distributions look very similar and suggest that the sample of 48 surgeons have workloads which match fairly closely the estimated workload of all British ophthalmologists.

In Figure 4.11 the trauma and orthopaedics estimated weekly average was 8.4 cases per week, and yet the actual figure in the sample shows only 4.6 cases per week. Whilst this might seem a significantly different result, it has to be remembered that in this

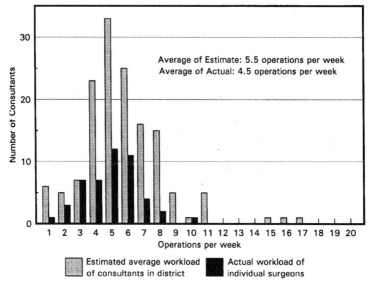

Figure 4.10   Actual and estimated weekly workloads in ophthalmology

Source:
Figures 4.2, 4.4

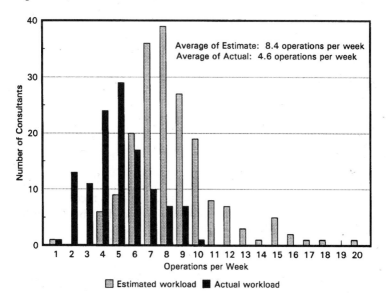

Figure 4.11   Actual and estimated weekly workloads in orthopaedics

Source:
Figure 4.4, IACC Time Series Indicators 1991–92

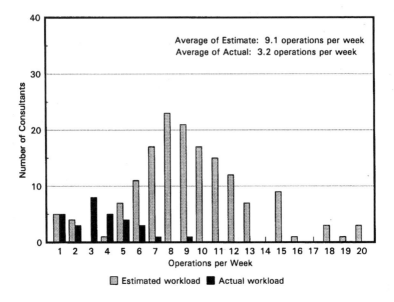

Figure 4.12 Actual and estimated weekly workloads in ENT

Source:
Figure 4.7, IACC Time Series Indicators 1991–92

specialty, junior surgeons actually undertook 57% of all operations in the actual workload category. If that figure was applied to the data for the whole of England, the estimated figure of an average of 8.4 would become 6.9 and the distributions would be closer together. Another explanation for the variation in the two distributions is that the sample examined is atypical. The fact that it relates to hospitals which had some of the worst waiting lists in the country might, in part, explain some of the difference.

In ENT the two distributions are enormously different. It seems quite clear that the set of 30 ENT surgeons studied, by any standards, had an exceptionally low workload. (Fig. 4.12).

Comparing the sample with a similar study

In 1994, the Audit Commission undertook a major study of the medical profession and as part of that study examined the activity of consultant surgeons (Audit Commission 1995). The selection of hospitals they chose to study was made on the basis of the operating theatre suites which had a computerized informa-

Table 4. 9   Operations per consultant per week

Specialty	Number of surgeons in study		Average number of operations per week	
	IACC	Audit Commission	IACC	Audit Commission
Trauma and orthopaedics	120	20	4. 6	4.6
Ophthalmology	48	8	4.4	6.4
ENT surgery	30	15	3.2	4.5
General surgery	15	28	7.2	5.6
Urology	4	12	7.4	9.7
Gynaecology	4	30	6.2	6.1

Sources:
IACC studies of specialties in British health authorities from 1989-1994
Audit Commission studies for The doctors' tale: the work of hospital doctors in
England and Wales (Audit Commission 1995)

tion system which recorded the name of the operating surgeon.
They studied all work from 8.00 a.m. to 6.00 p.m. for a group of
over 100 surgeons in 6 specialties. The results for those specialties
are displayed in Table 4.9 and show that for 5 specialties the
average number of operations per week was 4, 5 or 6 patients.
Only in urology was there an average of nearly 10 cases per
week. In 2 specialties, the Audit Commission figures were lower
than those arrived at in our own study.

SUMMARIZING THE EVIDENCE

In conclusion, it is difficult to argue that the sample of 274
surgeons is completely atypical of British surgical performance.
In ENT surgery it may be that the sample studied was rather
unusual, but in other specialties the array of activity appears to
be commensurate with any estimate that can be made of consultant surgeons' activity.

NHS managers have difficulty in accessing information about
the workload of their surgeons in the NHS and they have no
access to information on what surgeons do in the private sector.
This study of over 5% of British surgeons gives some insight into
consultant activity in the NHS. It shows that one-fifth of the
consultants in the sample undertook 3 or fewer operations per
week and spent surprisingly little time in the operating theatre.

The majority of consultant surgeons undertake 4, 5 or 6 operations per week and probably spend between 6 and 8 hours per week operating. This means that over two-thirds of their working week is dedicated to ward rounds, pre- and postoperative care, out-patient clinics, teaching, research and administration. The operative workload in the NHS includes a small proportion of private patients in NHS paybeds, but in the absence of any controlling mechanism, the NHS does not know whether any of its surgeons undertake a large proportion of their private operations in their own time or whether they do it in NHS time.

Is the NHS getting value for money from its surgeons? It may surprise the public to find that their average surgeon personally does 5 operations per week and spends as little as 6 to 8 hours of a 35-hour contracted week, operating in an NHS theatre. This seems a very low level of operating in the light of the fact that bonuses were offered to orthopaedic surgeons at the private Health Care International Hospital in Glasgow for doing 10 operations a day (Gillard 1994). Non-surgeons will need some convincing that the balance between operating and all the other in-patient tasks has been correctly set in the NHS. Is there some sort of restrictive practice being operated by managers and surgeons? Is the average volume of work low because the NHS does not provide surgeons with adequate resources, or do surgeons spend too much time playing golf or undertaking private practice? It is time for surgeons and managers in the NHS to start examining working practices and to gather data that in the past they have been loathe to study. Surgeons and managers must now demonstrate that the evidence presented here is substantially inaccurate, or else justify to the public that it is reasonable for highly trained surgeons to undertake an average of only 4 to 6 operations per week.

A tale of two cities?

In the second city, half of the operations are done by junior surgeons who do most of the emergency surgery. Consultants are contracted to spend most of their time in the city, but even so undertake only four or five operations per week. The consultants do not appear to get the opportunity to do more work. Whilst their work patterns are agreed with managers, the agreements appear minimalist and combined with the constraints in resources provided, means that the service given to the citizens in the second city is restricted.

TIME SPENT IN THE PRIVATE SECTOR

Whilst we are poorly informed about what surgeons do in the NHS, we are almost totally ignorant about what they do in the private sector. There are no systematic records which give details about their workload, or the amount of time they spend in the private hospitals and consulting rooms. There would be less interest in this subject if it were not for the fact that they are legally permitted to work both in the private sector and the NHS. Given the evidence in the previous chapter about the apparent constraints on operating time in the NHS, the curiosity is even greater about how much time is spent, by whom, and at what time of day, in the private sector.

WORKING TO THE LETTER OF THE CONTRACT?

Before we examine this question in detail, it is important to recognize that the casual observer can be easily drawn into unjustified criticism of the medical profession if he or she does not have knowledge of individual surgeons' contractual positions. No criticism can be levelled at a surgeon spending 3 or 4 half-days in private hospitals and rooms, if he is on a part-time contract and only obliged to spend 6 half-days working in the NHS. These part-time contracts are not common, but it is important to note that they do exist.

Surgeons with NHS contracts have both practical and contractual limits on the time they can devote to private practice. The practical constraints are that a senior NHS post is a demanding and strenuous appointment, with responsibilities that fill most of the working week. It also demands that surgeons are on call (and called) at evenings and weekends. Some would argue that those commitments are so arduous it is difficult to see how time can be made available for any other professional activity. Others would argue that many individuals have sufficient energy to work long hours and that the regular out of hours commitments to the NHS, combined with a flexible contract, enable surgeons to do private operating and consulting during the working week and still more than adequately cover their NHS duties and responsibilities. In recent times there has been the additional complication that restrictions on NHS activity imposed by resource constraints now leave some surgeons with more time to work in the private sector. Despite this increased freedom, the practical constraints alone would suggest that private practice is the minor part of surgeons' activity. It is generally assumed to be squeezed into free time available during the normal NHS working day or, more frequently, at the beginning and end of the working day.

In an earlier chapter I described how contractual limits have never been very clearly defined. The vast majority of consultant surgeons have maximum part-time contracts with the NHS. Both the NHS and the medical profession have always acknowledged that there is a need for some flexibility in hours of work because of the need for on-call commitments. In 1990, the Public Accounts Committee was assured that the newly introduced 'job plans' for consultants would be carefully monitored under the new management arrangements being introduced in the NHS. These required managers and surgeons to agree what duties a consultant would be routinely undertaking on 5 to 7 committed half-days per week. For a surgeon these 'hard' sessions would generally comprise half-days in operating theatres and out-patient clinics. A typical timetable for an orthopaedic surgeon is shown in Figure 5.1.

The remaining 'soft' sessions are to cover more variable activities. These would include ward rounds, teaching, research, audit, administration and travel, all of which are variable in terms of time. The job plans also require surgeons to specify the average number of hours spent on NHS activities, in both 'hard' and 'soft' sessions. Table 5.1 shows the list presented by one

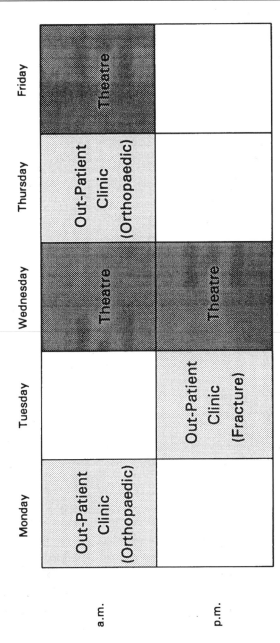

Figure 5.1 Typical timetable plan for an orthopaedic surgeon

	Monday	Tuesday	Wednesday	Thursday	Friday
a.m.	Out-Patient Clinic (Orthopaedic)		Theatre	Out-Patient Clinic (Orthopaedic)	Theatre
p.m.		Out-Patient Clinic (Fracture)	Theatre		

Table 5.1 Weekly duties of a consultant orthopaedic surgeon

Hours	Type of duty
10	Out-patients
5	Ward work
9	Theatre or special procedures
2	Teaching, training and examination
3	Research
1	Medical audit
1	Management
1	Committees, local or national
5	Administration
3	Travelling time

orthopaedic surgeon. Note that operating time is restricted to 9 hours per week and is less than the total spent on management, administration, committees and travelling. This surgeon also claims 3 hours per week are devoted to research, but it is very difficult for managers to check whether such commitments are honoured. In this case, the surgeon had not published a single research paper in any listed medical or scientific journal for at least 8 years.

Job plans differ between specialties and between surgeons within a specialty. Private practice is not normally shown on job plans, and is assumed to be slotted into one of the 'soft' half-days on the job plan, or done out of hours. Figure 5.2 sets out the typical elements of a working week in three specialties. It artificially shows the 'hard' sessions (operating lists and out-patient clinics) portrayed in the early part of each week and the 'soft' sessions at the end of the week. The fact that about 40% of the working week is classified in 'soft' half days and that 'flexibility' is written into the contract to take account of on-call and emergency work, means that consultants have some choice as to when they undertake their private practice. Most surgeons get into a pattern of holding regular 'rooms' sessions in the private sector on a nominated half-day, but operating is not necessarily done on such a regular basis. Most surgeons inform their NHS secretaries of their private commitment and there is no secret made of 'rooms' availability to either hospital staff, general practitioners or prospective patients.

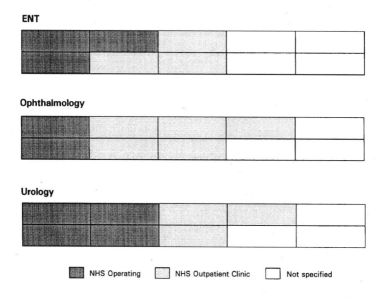

Figure 5.2   Elements of a working week in three specialties

Note Each cell represents 1 half-day

Whilst the existence of private practice is not secret, the effect on NHS patients is far from clear. This chapter attempts to shed some light on areas which to date have remained in the shadows. None of the methods used provide us with a complete understanding of the questions raised, but together they might establish a clearer picture. In the absence of routinely available data, we are left with:

- self-reported estimates of time by surgeons themselves
- estimates of time spent based on calculations made from studies of operations undertaken in the private sector
- surveys of availability for 'rooms' consultations
- observations of time spent in the private sector by sample individuals.

SELF-REPORTED INFORMATION

A survey of consultants' working hours was undertaken by the Monopolies and Mergers Commission (MMC) in their study of private medical services (1994a). 566 consultants responded to their interview survey. The largest group of 404 consultants held maximum part-time contracts and, on average, they recorded 62 hours work each per week. Of these, 51 hours were spent in the NHS and 11 in private practice. The survey included consultants from all specialties, both medical and surgical. The majority of consultants recorded that they worked considerably 'longer hours than a typical white-collar worker, with a significant number working the equivalent of six 13-hour days a week.' The MMC examined the data reported, to see if they could identify any relationship between NHS working hours and private practice working hours. Clear patterns were difficult to identify. Some of the consultants who worked long hours in the private sector were amongst those who also worked long hours in the NHS. These individuals appeared to support the theory that, if you want something done, you go to the busy person.

On the other hand, there were groups of consultants whose time spent in the private sector was equally as long and yet their commitment to the NHS was much less apparent. 70% of the consultants surveyed said they had no difficulty in fitting their private practice in with their NHS commitments. If the figures reported in this survey are accurate and reflect what consultant surgeons do in the NHS, it does suggest that the proportion of time spent undertaking NHS surgery is even lower than we had previously calculated. According to my calculations, surgeons spent about 6–11 hours operating out of a 35-hour contract week, whereas the MMC report suggests it is out of a 51-hour week. This means that their personal operating time is as little as 10–25% of their working week and that they devote over 40 hours per week to non-operative duties.

The MMC survey showed that an average of 11 hours per week was spent by consultants in private practice. However, over half of the consultants recorded less than 9 hours per week working in the private sector, and the vast majority of those spending in excess of 15 hours per week on private practice usually held less than maximum part-time contracts or were retired. Self-reported surveys do not suggest excessive times spent in the private sector by full-time or maximum part-time NHS surgeons.

ESTIMATING OPERATING TIME SPENT IN THE PRIVATE SECTOR

Some of the information published by, and about, the private sector gives us an indication of the volume of consultant activity and time spent in the private sector. *Laing's Review of Private Healthcare* (1993) lists the number of private hospitals and operating theatres in Britain. A Norwich Union study (Laing 1992a) examined the use of operating theatres in the private sector. Professor Brian Williams and his colleagues have undertaken three major studies of the level of activity in the private sector in England and Wales in 1981 (Nicholl et al 1984), 1986 (Nicholl et al 1989) and 1992–93 (Williams & Nicholl 1994). None of these studies, nor any other published information, tell us what individual surgeons do in the private sector, but we can begin to assess the total scale of such activity and how it might affect the weekly workload of consultant surgeons.

In 1993 there were at least 447 operating theatres in British private hospitals (*Laing's Review of Private Health Care* 1993). It is difficult to imagine that these would be built to be used only at weekends and in the evenings and, in any case, the Norwich Union study (Laing 1992a) reports that 72% of private sector operations take place between 9.00 a.m. and 5.00 p.m. on weekdays. A modest assumption would be that the private sector would endeavour to use the theatres for at least half of the working week. If the 429 theatres in England and Wales were used for 5 half-days per week each, to operate on 3 patients each half-day, this would add up to over 300 000 patients per year. It would also mean that each week over 2000 half-days of operating would be needed – more than enough to utilize 1 session a week for each anaesthetist and 1 session every 2 weeks for each surgeon.

In reality, the number of operations per year in the private sector is around 600 000. A survey of short-stay independent hospitals in England and Wales in 1992–93 (Williams & Nicholl 1994) calculated that there were 678 703 in-patient and day-case patients treated during the year, although 78 000 of these appeared to undergo no operative procedure. We can estimate how much time surgeons spend operating in the private sector during the working day by taking the following steps.

1. Norwich Union's own publication (Laing 1992a) shows that in the hospitals they surveyed, 72% of operating took place

between 9.00 a.m. and 5.00 p.m. Monday to Friday. On this basis we can estimate that in England and Wales there were 432 000 operations undertaken in 1 year during normal working hours.

2. In order to convert the operations into estimated operating time, I have assumed the distribution of case mix is similar to that as surveyed by the Norwich Union study of private hospitals (Laing 1992a). In that study 5487 operations were estimated to have taken 6177 hours (Table 4.3 Chap. 4). This would suggest that the 432 000 operations are likely to take somewhere between 485 000–500 000 hours per year of operating time in the private sector, during the working day.

3. In England and Wales in the same year there were 4626 consultant surgeons of various disciplines and 2342 consultant anaesthetists. Not all of these consultants undertook private practice, but as the majority did so, we can divide the number of hours spent in the private sector by the total number of surgeons to derive an *underestimate* of the number of hours per year per consultant spent in the private sector. For consultant surgeons the number of hours would be 105 per year and for consultant anaesthetists 207 per year.

4. If we assume a 46-week working year, the average surgeon would be spending a little over 2.3 hours per week operating in the private sector and anaesthetists just over 4.5 hours per week.

This calculation, which suggests that surgeons undertake about two operations per week in the private sector, was confirmed in a separate independent study undertaken by the Audit Commission (1995). This study of a group of over 100 surgeons and their work with two major insurers, covering 80% of the market, also revealed an average of two private operations per week. Given the exclusion of those patients who paid directly and 20% of the insured patients, an estimate of two cases per week seems to be a conservative figure.

Just as in the NHS, an average figure for private workload hides a wide range of activity. We know that there are some surgeons and anaesthetists who undertake no private practice, and we also know from the publications by Norwich Union (Laing 1992a) that there is a wide range of surgical activity per day in independent hospitals. Norwich Union themselves have published wide ranges of workload which show operating times from less than half an hour to well over 5 hours per day, and an income per surgeon ranging from under £250 to over £3000 per day. The Monopolies and Mergers Commission (1994a) pointed out that the top 10% of consultants accounted for 40% of the total gross private practice earnings in 1992 and in *The Lancet* it was stated that although two-thirds of consultants undertook both NHS and private work, 20% of the consultants carry out 66% of private work (Dean 1993).

From these calculations, it appears that the average NHS surgeon undertakes at least two private operations per week in independent hospitals during the working day. Given the need for immediate pre- and postoperative examination of patients and the fact that some travelling time will be necessary to reach the independent hospital, it is difficult to see how the average surgeon can manage two operations per week without committing the equivalent of one whole session per week to the private sector. Evidence suggests that for many surgeons the time spent will be much greater. It should also be noted that none of these calculations take any account of time spent in consulting rooms.

SURVEYS OF AVAILABILITY OF TIME FOR 'ROOMS' CONSULTATION IN THE PRIVATE SECTOR

Estimates of the potential availability of private consultations can be calculated by obtaining the out-patient and rooms schedules produced by some private hospitals for use by general practitioners or by direct enquiry to private hospitals and rooms. It must be recognized, however, that half-day availability on a regular basis does not automatically mean that the surgeon spends all of that time in the private hospital or rooms. In 1990, an enquiry into the amount of time spent by consultants in private rooms at the Priory Hospital in Birmingham (House of Commons Committee of Public Accounts 1990) found that both the employing authority and the consultants argued there was a distinction to be made between availability and actual attendance in the private sector:

Whilst consultants do have commitments to the private hospital, these are not usually fixed sessions, and the hours spent there are generally fewer than those suggested in the document circulated by the private hospital. No instance has been found where private commitments were undertaken to the detriment of the NHS, which, in fact, benefits from a significantly greater commitment by consultants than their formal contractual obligations would require.

In the light of this robust defence of surgeons by the NHS managers, I undertook a more detailed survey of rooms availability. I did not rely on the private hospitals' own published schedules, but made direct enquiries to the private secretaries of almost a quarter of England's trauma and orthopaedic surgeons. Towns and cities were selected to give complete geographical coverage of England. *The Medical Directory* (1993) was used to produce a list of surgeons working in each hospital in the towns, cities and sections of cities selected. Telephone calls to NHS secretaries were made to establish the rooms or private hospitals used by each surgeon, enquiries were made to private hospitals direct, and telephone directories were consulted. An enquiry was then made on behalf of a patient who was considering private surgery. Information was requested about:

- whether or not the consultant saw private patients
- the date of the next available appointment
- at what times during the week consultations were available and whether or not these times were available on a regular basis
- whether or not there were any vacancies available between the date of the telephone call and the next appointment given (to assess whether all sessions were regularly used).

I attempted to contact 183 trauma and orthopaedic surgeons. In six cases I was unable to obtain information. Of the 177 surgeons' secretaries contacted the availability for private consultation was as follows:

- 8 (5%) would not see private patients
- 12 (7%) would only see private patients outside normal working hours
- 68 (38%) set aside 1 half-day per week regularly for rooms consultation. This half-day was during the working week and was often supplemented by additional clinics at either lunchtimes, evenings or weekends
- 89 (50%) set aside 2 or more half-days for rooms consultations during the working week, some supplementing those clinics with additional out of hours sessions.

Rooms time alone accounted for at least 1 half-day per week for 88% of the orthopaedic surgeons studied. Half of the surgeons committed 2 or more half-days per week to rooms consultations.

This pattern of work was reasonably consistent across the country, although the private practice scene in London did seem to be somewhat different from the rest of the country. Of the 34 London surgeons included in the study, only 3 (9%) restricted private patient consultations to outside normal working hours, 9 (26%) set aside 1 half-day for rooms consultations and 22 (65%) set aside 2 or more half-days for rooms consultations. The tendency to undertake private rooms consultations during the working week was similar in London to elsewhere in England. Figure 5.3 shows quite clearly that regular rooms sessions during the working week is not a phenomenon restricted to the Harley Street and Wimpole Street area of London.

Similar surveys were undertaken in other specialties. In ophthalmology I selected two different groups of surgeons. The first set were those listed in *The Good Doctor Guide* (Page 1993) which lists doctors of many specialties, (mainly) in the London area. The guide claims to select specialists who are recommended by their colleagues. I assumed that most of these would undertake private practice, but that they would not be represen-

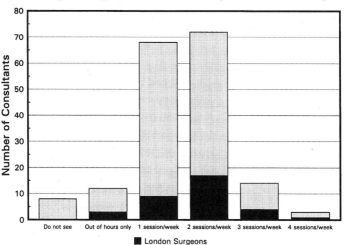

Figure 5.3 Survey of private rooms availability – 177 orthopaedic surgeons

Source:
IACC Survey September 1994

tative of normal British practice. The second set were ophthalmologists who were from district general hospitals and teaching hospitals outside London and who were likely to be much more representative of 'normal' practice.

There were 33 consultants listed in *The Good Doctor Guide* who were still practising at the time of my study. The average waiting time to see them in the private sector was 2½ weeks, with most consultants able to see private patients in 2 weeks or less. These surgeons devoted an average of 3 half-days per week to private rooms consultations and over a quarter gave 4 half-days per week to private rooms. We do not know what their contractual position was and some of them may have had part-time contracts. All held substantive NHS appointments and we can be sure that the majority held maximum part-time contracts that require them to devote substantially the whole of their time to the NHS.

The study of more 'normal' ophthalmologists outside London avoided the potential influence of Harley Street and Wimpole Street. This time I identified 37 ophthalmologists in towns throughout England with a mixture of specialist eye hospitals and ordinary district general hospitals. This list coincided with the English ophthalmologists referred to in an earlier chapter. The average waiting time for these consultants was less than 2 weeks and the average level of rooms availability was 2 half-days per week. Figure 5.4 shows the two groups of ophthalmologists. Whilst the provincial ophthalmologists spent less time in private rooms than their London counterparts, it is still quite clear that the norm for ophthalmologists is to spend 2, 3 or 4 half-days in rooms alone. Private operating time is additional to these figures.

These surveys demonstrate that private practice during the working day is a common occurrence. There may well be an argument, on the part of the medical profession, that not every rooms session is fully occupied (not supported by the evidence in this study) and that the surgeons do indeed do other work at other times in the NHS to compensate. However, the first loyalty of the surgeons during those sessions is to the private sector and only if not enough private patients turn up might the surgeon then decide to return to the NHS to which he is contracted to give priority at all times.

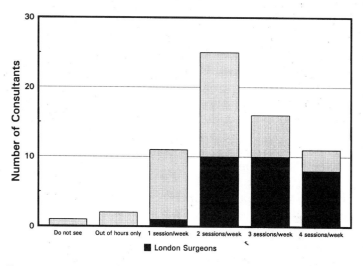

Figure 5.4   Survey of private rooms availability – 66 ophthalmic surgeons

Source:
IACC Survey September 1994

OBSERVATIONS OF TIME SPENT BY SAMPLE INDIVIDUALS

Occasionally, a newspaper or television report will announce that a consultant has fiddled his travelling expenses or broken one of the bureaucratic rules about the treatment of private patients in the NHS. All human endeavour results in some failure and this sort of misdemeanour, whilst regrettable, cannot be seriously classified as a major systems failure. More prevalent is the consistent anecdote and innuendo about the way senior medical and surgical staff are prepared to give a disproportionate amount of their time to private patients and how they inequitably allow those who have money to have undue priority over those who do not. Such innuendo and anecdote rarely appear in writing, and when they do, a closer examination seldom produces a cast iron case of abuse. Some of the examples that do occur tend to find their way into sensational media or politically extreme propaganda and the motivation behind publication is often seen as suspect. Rather than quote from such sources which tend to rely on second-hand stories with incomplete observation, I will illustrate the problem we face by using an example which I can vouch for personally. It was this example that originally alerted me to the potential magnitude of the inequality inherent in our health system.

In 1986, one consultant ophthalmologist could be seen by his NHS patients for a routine out-patient appointment only after a wait of 43 weeks. He and his team of juniors had, for a number of years, been operating on around 600 patients per annum. The majority of those patients were operated on at a main specialist hospital but 50–100 operations took place during a weekly operating session held at a nearby district general hospital. The patients who were operated on at the main specialist hospital were on one of two theatre lists. One was never attended by the consultant surgeon but was always undertaken by senior registrar or other junior staff. In 1986 the two operating lists at the main hospital involved 538 operations, of which 178 were undertaken by the surgeon himself and 368 by his juniors. Of the 178 patients operated on by the consultant surgeon, 82 were NHS patients and the remaining 96 were private patients. The consultant surgeon had a maximum part-time NHS contract for which he was paid ten-elevenths of a consultant's salary. His regular commitments to the NHS were as follows:

- one regular operating session in a main NHS hospital, in which half of his operating was on private patients
- one general out-patient clinic at the main hospital, which was huge and very busy, but, nevertheless, occasionally included one or two private patients
- one operating session per week at a nearby general hospital which averaged less than two operations per week
- a clinic at the nearby general hospital
- rounds to visit the patients on the wards, particularly at the main specialist hospital on up to three occasions per week
- a specialist clinic at the main hospital for patients with a particular condition; the numbers attending this clinic were very small and the consultant did not always attend for a full $3^1/_2$ hour session.

The consultant was routinely available in his private rooms for 4 half-day sessions each week. These facts were verified over a 2-year period by regular visits and telephone calls to the rooms and direct observation of the surgeon's arrival and departure times. However flexible the NHS contract, it seems difficult to interpret this man's work pattern as 'devoting substantially the whole of his time to the NHS' which is what his NHS contract required. This example raises three questions.

1. Is this an isolated and rare example?
2. Does this sort of thing no longer occur?
3. Is this pattern of behaviour only found in ophthalmology?

The medical profession denies there is a serious problem and NHS managers are unable to determine the position as they have no data collection system in place to answer our questions in the affirmative or negative. If a group of professionals state that they are doing more than a fair day's work for a day's pay and a substantial section of those around them, including managers, politicians and patients, accept that is the case, ought that not to be taken on face value? The fact that we have established that some surgeons have a low NHS workload might be explained by inadequate NHS resources. The fact that some surgeons appear to spend a large amount of time in the private sector, might be due to a lack of clarity of the contractual rules and a gross misinterpretation of what actually happens. In other words, the surveys of time spent in rooms and the calculations of how much time might be spent in operating theatres, are all error prone and do not actually reflect what individual surgeons do.

Perhaps the only way to establish a consultant's commitment to the NHS and the private sector would be to follow him for every minute of his working day and record each activity he undertakes. The trouble would be that, just like all of us, he would modify his behaviour if he knew he was being observed. If he is asked to self-record his activity he would no doubt be inclined to paint a rosy picture. (The same criticism applies to any self-recorded data collection.) We could determine a consultant's normal working pattern very accurately by observation without the consultant's knowledge. This type of surveillance offends most liberal thinking, but is nevertheless employed by society when abuse is suspected and when no other checking mechanism is in place. A well-known example of this is the employment of fraud officers by the DHSS, who follow benefit claimants to ensure they are not making false claims.

The evidence presented earlier in this chapter derived from estimates of operating time and surveys of private rooms availability provides a disturbing picture. It suggests that a high proportion of surgeons spend 2 or 3 half-days per week working in the private sector. I was concerned, however, that the picture painted was an over-exaggeration and I needed some mechanism for testing out my fears. The only way I could clarify this issue was to have a precise log of how consultants spend their time. Such a log is difficult to obtain and various methods of information collection were attempted to establish the normal weekly working pattern of a sample of consultants. These included telephoning and visiting all locations used by the consultant for a complete week and, having established the likely pattern of time spent in the private sector, then confirming those half-day sessions over a much longer period, in order to ensure that the selected week was not atypical.

The first method involved using a group of volunteer students and unemployed persons who formed an amateur 'detective agency'. During 1 year, 3 separate months were selected to study a group of specialists in four district health authorities. The volunteer group contacted all the NHS hospitals in the districts concerned and ascertained the names of the consultants in two specialties. Then, by enquiries through Hospital Records Departments, secretarial staff, NHS managers and telephone directories, the volunteers attempted to piece together the normal working pattern of each consultant.

During most of the first month, despite daily visits to all the locations, the volunteers found it difficult to identify precise routines for all consultants, but eventually some clear patterns became evident. Particularly clear patterns were easy to establish in terms of time spent in private rooms. Receptionists in the private sector are very willing to give full details of availability. As many rooms are in converted houses, with nameplates and car parks clearly visible from the road, it was easy to establish the working pattern of surgeons who made regular visits to those locations. Over 700 sightings were made during the 3-month period, together with hundreds of telephone calls. In a few instances, despite telephone calls and visits to all known NHS hospitals and all listed private hospitals and rooms over the 3-month period, some consultants were never located on some half-days. Whilst the method was clearly deficient in obtaining completely accurate information about consultants' timetables, it did, nevertheless, enable clear patterns to be identified for major parts of the week for some surgeons. An illustration of the type of log that could be prepared for each surgeon is shown in Table 5.2.

Table 5.2 Schedule of the weekly activity of one consultant surgeon

Day	Schedule	Confirmation of activity	% of time on private work
Monday a.m.	NHS operating	a) Analysis of theatre register b) Analysis of financial records	30
Monday p.m.	NHS special clinic	a) Telephoning NHS b) Direct observation c) Analysis of financial records	0
Tuesday a.m.	NHS operating	a) Analysis of theatre register b) Analysis of financial records	30
Tuesday p.m.	NHS operating	a) Analysis of theatre register b) Analysis of financial records	30
Wednesday a.m.	NHS clinic and research	a) Telephoning NHS b) Direct observation	0
Wednesday p.m.	Private rooms	a) Telephoning rooms b) Direct observation	100
Thursday a.m.	Private rooms	a) Telephoning rooms b) Direct observation	100
Thursday p.m.	NHS clinic	a) Telephoning NHS b) Direct observation c) Analysis of financial records	10
Friday a.m.	Private rooms	a) Telephoning rooms b) Direct observation	100
Friday p.m.	NHS clinic	a) Telephoning NHS b) Direct observation c) Analysis of financial records	0
Total % time on private work			40

From my point of view the results were unsatisfactory. Despite demonstrating that a consultant was present in his or her private rooms at 11.00 a.m. one morning, one cannot necessarily conclude that he or she was there for the whole of that morning. It could well be that on all the occasions where consultants were found to be in private rooms or private hospitals, they were only there for a short period of time and then quickly returned to the NHS. To produce irrefutable evidence a much fuller and more professional set of observations would be needed.

As a further check, I used research funds provided by a charitable trust to employ professional private detectives to verify the amateur observation results and calculations made in my research. Selecting a firm that had been used to undertake just such a study on behalf of a health authority, I provided the names of two groups of surgeons. One group was suspected of devoting a considerable amount of time to the private sector and the other group was thought to be dedicated almost exclusively to the NHS. The findings were depressing. The professional firm found that all the consultants in both groups spent some time in the private sector, but the group that we had suspected as spending a high proportion of time in the private sector (up to four sessions per week on maximum part-time contracts) did indeed do so.

The following four examples are typical of the findings revealed by various study methods. In the cases cited the evidence about the amount of time spent in the private sector is clear cut and it is absolutely certain that the surgeons concerned routinely spent at least 3 or 4 half-days a week working in the private sector.

1. An ENT surgeon who operates on 2 half-days each week at two different private hospitals. On neither of the half-days does he have any routine NHS commitment. He also has private rooms sessions on 2 other half-days each week. In addition, managers have recently expressed concern about the volume of private insurance work being undertaken in one of the NHS clinics.
2. An ophthalmologist who routinely commits 3 half-day sessions in his private rooms every week. He does not operate in the private sector, but chooses to place his private patients on NHS operating lists. In one NHS clinic he routinely sees one or two private patients each week.

3. A plastic surgeon who can be found working in the private sector for up to 2 whole days each week. His NHS schedule involves him visiting many NHS hospitals, but over a period of 8 weeks he was found to be working in a private hospital for, at least, some part of almost every working day. The average time spent in the private sector was never less than 4 half-days per working week.

4. A cardiac surgeon who did not appear in the NHS between 9.00 am and 5.00 p.m. on 2 whole days per week. Of this time, 3 half-days were spent in the private sector, and the remaining half-day was used to pursue other personal interests.

At the time the evidence was gathered, all four of these surgeons were on maximum part-time NHS contracts and all the evidence clearly suggests that this is the normal pattern of working throughout the whole year. Each of the four works in a different NHS health district and together they represent four of the major surgical specialties. In each case, similar information was obtained about the other surgeons working in the district in the specialty concerned, and, in each case, for all of the maximum part-time surgeons, there was routinely a minimum of 3 half-days per week spent in the private sector.

CUSTOM AND PRACTICE

The conclusion must be that most British surgeons are spending between 1 and 3 half-days per week in the private sector. There is a wide range of behaviour, with some surgeons spending no time at all in the private sector during normal working hours, whilst at the other extreme some could be devoting as much as half the working week to private sector activity. There are no accepted guidelines against which any monitoring can be compared and the vagueness of phrases such as 'devote substantially the whole of your time' and 'flexible agreement' leaves surgeons with considerable freedom of a sort seldom enjoyed by other professional groups. The evidence presented here suggests that the time spent in the private sector is excessive and might be outside the terms of an extremely vague contract. It is also quite clear that the optimism expressed by Sir Duncan Nichol and the NHS Management Executive that the newly created system of job plans would enable a closer monitoring of the situation than hitherto, was ill-founded. Sir Duncan Nichol's suggestion that only half a day per week would be spent in private practice is clearly a myth.

When I first started this work, I wondered how many surgeons would need to be studied for how many weeks and over how many years before politicians, managers and the medical profession would be prepared to admit that there is some genuine conflict between time spent in the NHS and time spent in the private medical sector. I now realize that proving how much time is spent in the private sector is not the issue. Everybody knows that a high proportion of time is spent in the private sector. The problem is that no-one is concerned about it. Custom and practice in the NHS allows surgeons to operate their contracts in a flexible manner, which is said to be to the advantage of the NHS. It is argued that time spent during the working day in the private sector is more than compensated for by long working hours and substantial periods of on-call cover at evenings and weekends.

Consultants themselves reported to the Monopolies and Mergers Commission (1994a) that they had an average working week of 62 hours. Of these hours, 11 were spent in the private sector, which meant that the NHS was getting 16 hours extra on top of expected contract hours. On this basis it seems a small price to pay to allow your consultants to work for 11 hours in the private sector, if they give you an extra 16 hours in return. It might seem a little churlish to suggest precisely how many half-days of the normal working week ought to be spent in the NHS.

The BMA and the medical profession have never accepted the guidance suggested by Sir Duncan Nichol, that surgeons should only spend 1 half-day per week in the private sector, and regard his statement to the Public Accounts Committee on 22 January 1990 as incorrect or ill-informed. The current interpretation of job plans appears to be that consultants can legitimately spend 2, 3 or 4 half-days per week working in the private sector, without compromising their NHS contract.

A tale of two cities?

In the first city there are virtually no junior surgeons. The citizens are served by consultants who are mainly contracted to work in the second city. The consultants sometimes operate on weekday evenings and at weekends, but more frequently find time to operate during the working day. Despite contracts which require them to devote substantially the whole of their time to the second city, they routinely spend a day and a half per week in the first city.

6

Piecing together the jigsaw

PUTTING THE EVIDENCE IN ORDER

In front of me are the files of evidence I have gathered together over the past few years. They are like pieces of a jigsaw in jumbled piles all over the table. As I try to piece them together, I realize that they might not all be from the same jigsaw, but there seem to be common threads that run through different pictures. Some pieces appear to be of a background of uncertainty and lack of clarity. In the middle distance is a partially hidden and somewhat sinister area of inefficiency and in the foreground is a stark picture of imbalance and inequality. The re-arranged order becomes easier to follow (Table 6.1). Although I have not got all the pieces, it seems as if there may be one picture for each

Table 6.1 Are there inks between health care systems and inequitable access to health care?

Background of uncertainty	1. Considerable surgical discretion
	2. Weak contractual control
Areas of inefficiency	3. Some low volumes in NHS surgery
	4. High volume private surgery by some surgeons
	5. Regular private rooms sessions in working day
Resulting inequality?	6. High proportion of planned surgery for paying patients
	7. Length of waiting time determined by ability to pay

specialty. I begin to see a link between the health care system that we have in this country and the inequality faced by the patients in that system. Let us look at each pile of evidence, in the order shown in Table 6.1, before trying to complete some of the jigsaws.

Surgical discretion

The third chapter of this book examined the level of clinical discretion enjoyed by surgeons. The BMA has argued that it is time for ministers, patients' representatives and philosophers to join the medical profession in building a consensus and re-drawing the boundaries of NHS treatment. The rationing of health care is now regarded as a fact of life, and doctors of all disciplines face difficult choices over which patients to treat. The BMA Chairman (Lee-Potter 1995) has argued: 'clear guidelines must be agreed to bring consistency to decisions on medical and surgical priorities throughout the Health Service. We will never have enough resources to meet demand.' The position is actually more complex than that, because it is not simply a case of trying to cope with what is seen as an infinite demand, but also finding a way through a maze of inappropriate surgical and medical procedures. Decisions on the rationing of health care are exceptionally difficult to make when there is so much conflicting evidence about the scientific appropriateness of much of health treatment.

Set in the two different cultures of the NHS and the private sector, decision-making becomes even more difficult for the surgeons. A surgeon friend of mine has argued that the greatest area of ethical and moral dilemma in his life was that of trying to make similar and fair decisions in the two systems. He felt there was a grave danger that discretion meant saying yes to the rich and no to the poor. Surgical discretion is wide enough to be abused by those who wish to do so. Surgeons who work in both sectors run the risk of adopting double standards. I have met ophthalmologists who refused to share an NHS operating theatre with surgeons of another discipline because of the dangers of cross infection. They argued bitterly that they were not prepared to allow the NHS to compromise patients' safety. Nonetheless, they would happily walk into the neighbouring private hospital and undertake operations in a theatre suite shared with the same surgeons of other disciplines whom they had refused to allow near their own NHS theatres. Surgical discretion needs to be bounded by scientific considerations rather than personal whims.

Apathy about the conflicts of interest

The second chapter of this book traces the history of apathy over a contract which enables consultants to work for two competing employers. Much of the evidence assembled relates to consultants on maximum part-time contracts and it was these contracts that managers found most difficult to monitor. There has, however, been little evidence that their monitoring of full-time employees fared much better.

Surgeons and anaesthetists who hold full-time contracts are not permitted to earn more than 10% of their NHS salary in the private sector in 3 consecutive years without changing their contract to a maximum part-time contract. An anaesthetist friend of mine told me that he had put both his sons through private school on the fees he had earned by anaesthetizing in his local private hospital. Throughout that period he had held a full-time NHS contract and could not possibly have paid for two lots of school fees from a sum that was less than 10% of his NHS salary. Either he had another source of income he had not told me about, or he had not declared the true extent of private sector earnings to his NHS employers. When I started work on the

National Waiting List Initiative I came across a small 34-bed private hospital that had at least 11 full-time anaesthetists and a greater number of full-time surgeons on its books. The hospital routinely ran operating sessions during the normal working day and must have used some of these full-time NHS staff at times when they should have been working in the NHS. NHS managers simply do not monitor this type of activity.

One of the reasons why managers find it difficult to challenge surgeons about the dilemmas of the private sector–NHS interface is that they share exactly the same dilemma. In order to obtain revenue for their hospitals, chief executives often negotiate private patient contracts in NHS facilities. This sometimes causes tension and there are examples of private patient contracts having to be completed in sessions that would normally be used for NHS patients, thus either lengthening the NHS waiting list or requiring NHS patients to be operated on at weekends, and at more expense.

Recent moves to place consultants' contracts with local trusts, rather than regional health authorities, is likely to lead to a further deterioration in what was already a quite inadequate mechanism to deal with disciplinary problems amongst senior medical staff. Donaldson's study (1994) of one English region described 96 different types of problems that occurred in the disciplining of senior medical staff, including a lack of commitment to duties, some of which were explicitly linked to private practice. He pointed out: 'Dealing with such problems requires experience, objectivity, and a willingness to tolerate unpleasantness and criticism. Because most consultants' contracts are now held by NHS Trust hospitals, however, those who had developed a skill over the years in handling these complex issues are now no longer involved.' Neither doctors nor managers have any incentive to demarcate between NHS and private sector activity. Those surgeons who are dedicated to the NHS find increasing difficulty in arranging meetings about NHS business or clinical research, because their colleagues are so committed to the private sector.

Low-volume operating in the NHS

The fourth chapter of this book tried to ascertain how many operations are performed by NHS surgeons in NHS hospitals. At that point I briefly mentioned that not all of the operating done in the

NHS is on NHS patients. Since its inception in 1948 the NHS has always allowed the admission of private patients, who pay the surgeon for undertaking the operation and the National Health Service for the use of theatres, beds and other facilities in the hospital. The proportion of private patients receiving treatment in NHS hospitals has never been great and even in 1992–93 represented less than 2.5% of all elective surgery in the NHS.

The overall position, however, hides pockets of substantial use of NHS theatres for private patients. Some surgeons prefer to treat their private patients in an NHS hospital and there is little managerial control over this activity.

- In a specialist centre for plastic surgery, during a 13-week period, consultants operated on 218 patients, of whom 62 were private. One of the surgeons admitted only 8 private patients out of 61, whilst one of his colleagues admitted 40 private patients out of 76.
- In a large district general hospital in the East of England an orthopaedic surgeon personally operated on 1 private patient for every 3 NHS patients on his NHS operating lists.
- In a hospital in the North of England an ophthalmologist had a similar proportion of private to NHS work for his total workload – but his juniors were doing much of the NHS work.
- An ophthalmologist in a major teaching centre operated on 45 cases in 13 weeks, but two-thirds of the operations were keratotomies, (an operation which means a patient need no longer wear spectacles), which most regard as a low-priority cosmetic operation frequently conducted on private patients.
- In Northern Ireland there is only one hospital that undertakes cardiac surgery and yet in that NHS hospital 11% of all patients operated on are private. The information was disclosed as a result of a Parliamentary question (Ancram 1994), but despite there being enormous waiting lists in the province for heart surgery, no managerial, political or patient group interest seemed to be generated by the fact that an NHS facility had its capacity reduced significantly because it was taking private patients.
- In a London teaching hospital a consultant admitted 60 patients for cardiac surgery in 7 weeks, of whom 11 were private. Private operations were routinely undertaken, not only on Saturday mornings, but also on Wednesdays.

Hospital managers do not show any concern over the balance of private and NHS operating in the NHS. An increase in private patients means increased income for the hospital, so they condone and even encourage a growing number of private admissions at the expense of NHS patients. There is also a suspicion that the level of private practice may be under-recorded in the NHS. Theatre registers rarely record the status of patients and there is no automatic mechanism for comparing financial records with theatre records.

The examples above merely illustrate that for a small number of individual surgeons, the workload in the NHS is not all that it seems to be. A few of them choose to use the system to their own advantage, but this does not imply, let alone prove, that a large proportion of surgeons abuse the system. The vast majority of operating undertaken by most consultant surgeons in the NHS is on NHS patients.

The main conclusion in Chapter 4 was that many consultant surgeons undertake only four, five or six operations per week. Few have more than three operating sessions in which to do that work and, given the widely perceived need for many surgical operations, the actual level of operating appears low. It might be interesting to analyse consultant job plans throughout the country to discover how many surgeons spend less than a quarter of their NHS time in operating theatres and yet give over a third of their time to an assortment of duties that have little direct benefit on patient care. The failure of NHS managers to obtain more surgery from surgeons is widely attributed to inadequate resource provision. Underfunding and inefficiency are a potent cocktail that does not serve the patient well.

Operating in the private sector

Chapter 5 estimated how many operations consultants undertook during the working day in private hospitals. It could be argued that the calculations were based on sample surveys and statistics and that they do not reflect the situation in all private hospitals up and down the land. In the absence of detailed information on operating theatre usage in every private hospital in the country, it is difficult to take the debate much further until this anomaly is rectified. I can, however, observe what happens to my neighbours and friends. Living as I do in an affluent conurbation, I have many friends who work in private hospitals and even more friends who are operated on in those hospitals. The great majority of those who have been admitted for an operation have had that operation during the normal working day, and theatre sisters, anaesthetists and surgeons all tell me that their private theatres are extremely busy on most working days.

Page (1993) argued that the volume of private surgery in London is enormous, and that foreigners alone are currently estimated to spend over £1 billion per year on treatment. 'Most foreign patients are from continental Europe. In 1993, at least three NHS surgical teams, while working privately part-time, in American-owned private hospitals in central London, each carried out more open heart operations on Europeans of other nationalities than all those undertaken on Finns in Finland.' He doesn't actually say how many operations are undertaken in Finland, but the implication is that the volume of work in London is extremely high. Page is indeed concerned about the risks of surgeons doing too much work. 'Surgeons leave home on Monday at 6.30 a.m. ... there is a macho ethic of never being tired. This is the danger posed to NHS and private patients alike.' He is probably wrong. For once, the poor and the NHS may have a real advantage.

Time spent in private rooms

Chapter 5 demonstrated the amount of time many surgeons spend in their private sector rooms. I first realized this might be a problem when we came across an ophthalmologist who never used one of his NHS theatre sessions. I was discussing this with one of my colleagues who, by chance, had taken a friend to see the very same surgeon the previous week. It was then we realized why he was not in his NHS theatre – that particular afternoon was one of his routine weekly sessions in his private rooms. Little data has been gathered about the use of rooms in the private sector. Some surgeons tell me that today over half the patients they see in their rooms pay cash and are not insured. Patients see this as a perfectly legitimate way of jumping the first half of the waiting list queue and many people in our society can afford a £50–£70 consulting fee. In theory, such patients should be placed on the NHS in-patient waiting list on the date they would have been seen in an NHS out-patient clinic (Department of Health and Social Security 1986) but this regulation is difficult to fulfil and even more difficult to monitor. Whilst there are examples of surgeons allowing patients to jump the first half of the queue by this method, we have little idea of the extent of this activity.

Over the last 2 years, since the introduction of general practitioner fundholders, there is now beginning to be anecdotal evidence of cash payments being made to consultants from fundholding GPs, either for seeing patients in the GP surgeries or, alternatively, in private hospitals. One wonders how long it will be before we return to the pre-1948 'fee splitting' arrangements whereby GPs were said to profit from a 'kick back' from the fees paid to surgeons by patients.

Disproportionate volumes of surgery

In the first chapter we examined the apparently unfair balance between the volume of surgery in the NHS and private sector. The work of Williams and Nicholl (1994) suggested that a fifth of all routine surgery was likely to be undertaken on private patients by 1991–92. It has subsequently been suggested that in some places this figure may now be as high as 40% (Devlin 1994).

It is also clear that at least half of the operating done in this country in the NHS is undertaken by juniors, and thus the proportion of the consultant's own work in the private sector will be even higher. For example, if a consultant does 20 operations in the private sector and his team does 80 operations in the NHS, then the proportion of private work overall is 20%. If, however, 40 of the 80 NHS operations are done by junior surgeons, then the proportion of the consultant's private operating is 33% (i.e. 20 private operations out of 60 operations in total).

The moral dilemma that faces both managers and surgeons is that their ethical codes of conduct actually challenge the very concept of private health care – that those who are prepared to pay can receive speedy treatment and priority over NHS patients. The Institute of Health Services Management has a statement of values which it expects its members to adhere to (undated). They should: 'Strive for accessible and effective health care according to need.' The British Medical Association took a firm stance over equity of access to the NHS, when it discovered that fundholder GPs were 'fast-tracking' – obtaining treatment more quickly for their patients than other patients with the same or greater need, but who were patients of GPs who were not fundholders. So strongly did the BMA feel about this issue that when in dispute with the government over the question of locally negotiated pay scales, they argued that 'consultants would insist on treating all patients on the basis of clinical need' (Beecham 1994b). Patients should be comforted by the BMA's firm stance, although perhaps a little disappointed to see that it is taken only when pay negotiations are in some difficulty and apparently does not apply to the treatment of private patients, who continue to be treated on the basis of ability to pay. The Royal College of Surgeons has as its motto the phrase 'Skills for the benefit of all men'. Perhaps this should be updated by adding 'provided they have the money'.

Inequality of waiting times

At the start of my research I was struck by the contrast in waiting times that confronted some of my friends and neighbours. In case there was some peculiar phenomena about the locality in which I lived, I surveyed NHS and private waiting times across the whole of the country, only to confirm that the discrepancies I had observed in my own neighbourhood were indeed widespread. As my research developed a television director friend took an increasing interest in what I was doing. As a professional journalist, he challenged the evidence I was putting forward and he sent a TV researcher to check out the stories of my friends, neighbours and professional colleagues. The researcher's job was to discover whether indeed there were such discrepancies in waiting time between the NHS and the private sector.

Within a very short time, stories similar to those I have heard time after time for 20 years came to the surface. People in my own church stepped forward with current examples of how they or their relatives were having to wait for treatment or pay to jump the queue. A mother showed an appointment card for her daughter who was offered a 54-week wait to see an orthopaedic surgeon. Another mother faced by the same dilemma had decided to pay privately to see the surgeon because on a previous occasion the lump on her daughter's leg had needed urgent surgery. The local newspaper was running a story of another mother who, with the help of her local pub, was raising money to ensure that her son's leg-lengthening operation could be done more speedily. Elderly folk and those who work with them came forward with examples of waiting months for cataract surgery and hip replacements. A recently retired fireman with a bladder problem was offered a 9-month wait to see the local urologist. A general practitioner produced a letter confirming that one of his patients requiring surgery did indeed have to wait over a year for an out-patient appointment. The registrar kindly informed him, in writing, that the only way to speed up the process was for the patient to go privately or to transfer to a fundholding GP, who would be able to get an earlier appointment.

I had assumed that these problems of inequality in waiting time would be restricted to those needing planned surgery for non-life threatening conditions, but it proved not to be the case. A policeman's wife with a lump on her breast found that she needed to use the private sector to get an early opinion on whether or not she had carcinoma – a decision which was coloured by the death of a young friend only 2 weeks earlier, who had had the same symptoms. General practitioners claimed that patients were now paying to have barium meals (a diagnostic procedure) and that private practice is now an option that has to be considered for urgent cases and not just for planned surgery.

The problem is not restricted to my own locality. A cutting from the *London Evening Standard* (Ghouri 1994) describes how a young women had spent $23^1/_2$ hours in a casualty department waiting to be admitted to a bed. During the process she had enquired about the possibility of a private bed and 'within 10 minutes a smiling ward manager appeared, application in hand. Yes, of course I could have a private bed immediately at the small cost of £270 per night plus treatment. Just fill in the form.' The young woman went on, 'I began to cry. There was no way I could possibly afford it.'

THREE SIMILAR PICTURES

This sequence of evidence does not prove that an inequitable distribution of waiting time is caused by allowing surgeons to work for both the state and the private sector, but the consistency with which common threads occur does raise the question of whether the relationship between the two is cause and effect.

However, simply to identify a group of surgeons who undertake very few operations in the NHS and also have long out-patient waiting times does not mean that those two problems are caused by the surgeons spending a large proportion of their time in the private sector. It could just as easily be caused by the fact that the NHS fails to give those surgeons sufficient resources to do the job properly. The evidence presented so far in this chapter has merely grouped the issues. A clearer picture emerges when we assemble evidence about individual specialties. Using the framework outlined in Table 6.1, let us look at how the evidence fits in three specialties.

THE ENT JIGSAW

The ENT specialty dominates the care of the ear, nose and throat and includes serious head and neck cancer work. There is some overlap with other specialties and it is quite common, for example, for plastic surgeons to undertake the same or similar nose operations as ENT surgeons.

Surgical discretion

For most of this century the specialty has been dominated by operations to remove tonsils and adenoids. At one stage this constituted two-thirds of all the specialty's operations, but today represents about one-third. The steady decline in the annual number of operations performed was arrested 3 years ago, when the number began to increase – possibly in response to the pressure to reduce waiting lists. The precise content of waiting lists by condition is not known, but surveys have suggested that over half of ENT waiting lists are made up of patients awaiting tonsil and adenoid removal. There is little agreement about the criteria for deciding whether the operation is actually necessary, and throughout this century there have been very wide variations in operation rates that are most likely to be explained by differences in surgical opinion, rather than any other variable. Throughout the history of the operation there has been disagreement about how appropriate the procedure is, and it is even claimed that over half of the operations carried out need never have been performed.

In the late 1980s, when the overall level of tonsil removal was reducing, there appeared to be an epidemic of 'glue ear' operations, a procedure for which there are similar doubts regarding appropriateness. This operation is now the second most common ENT operation. Together, tonsil and adenoid removal and operations for glue ear constitute over half of all ENT operations.

Contractual issues

ENT consultant surgeons are usually expected to do 3 operating sessions and 3 out-patient clinics per week. The 3 operating lists combined provide about 10–11 hours operating time per week, but this has to be shared with junior staff who may perform over half of the operations carried out. Some consultants are not even given 3 operating lists per week and many surgeons are likely to spend less than 5 hours per week personally operating, out of a contracted 35-hour week. Consultants claim the actual amount of time they spend in the NHS exceeds 50 hours per week, although in ENT there are no substantial on-call commitments to operate at weekends or in the evenings. Managers have little information about what ENT surgeons actually do in the 4 half-day sessions per week not committed to operating or out-patient clinics.

NHS volume

Data is not publicly available about the workload of individual surgeons, and NHS managers do not know how many operations each consultant ENT surgeon does. Given that there are 429 ENT consultants in England and Wales and that in England alone there are over 300 000 NHS operations per year, each consultant is likely to be responsible for about 16–18 operations per week in a working year of 46 weeks. If half of all operations are done by juniors, consultant ENT surgeons average 8–9 operations per week in the NHS. Some of these may be on private patients using NHS facilities, and half of them are likely to be tonsil and adenoid or glue ear operations.

Two studies have been conducted, which together have surveyed the work of 45 consultant ENT surgeons, providing a 10% sample of consultant activity. The 15 ENT surgeons studied by the Audit Commission (1995) revealed an average of 4.5 operations per week per consultant and the study of 30 ENT consultants reported in Chapter 4 found an average of only 3.2 cases per week with no fully qualified ENT surgeon doing more than 7 per week. The only known example of a consultant's personal workload being made public was as the result of the surgeon contracting the HIV virus (Clouston 1994). It was reported that the surgeon had undertaken 700 operations in 10 years, representing little more than 2 per week even assuming a 40-week year. There is no way of knowing whether these 46 surgeons are atypical of ENT consultants.

Private sector operating

In 1992–93 it is estimated there were 13 000 tonsil and adenoid operations and 32 000 other ENT operations carried out in independent hospitals in England and Wales. This would mean that the average ENT surgeon performs 2 private operations per week in independent hospitals. The distribution of private work between individual surgeons is likely to be very wide as there are some ENT surgeons who do no private operating, and others (on maximum part-time contracts) who routinely have 2 private operating sessions per week.

Rooms commitments

No information is available about the use of rooms by ENT surgeons.

Balance of surgery

In 1981, 14. 5% of tonsils and adenoids operations were done in the private sector, despite the fact that only 7.3% of the population were privately insured. By 1986 the percentages were 16.2% and 9% respectively. No more recent data has been produced for the proportion of operations undertaken on private patients, although the proportion of the population privately insured had increased to 11% by 1991–92. The fact that the majority of ENT operations are performed on children may mean that comparing operation rates with the insured population (mainly adult) may not be appropriate.

The sample of 45 ENT consultants showed that an average of

between 3.2 and 4.5 operations per week were performed in the NHS. The average in the private sector was calculated as 2 per week. These figures might suggest that as many as 30–40% of consultant ENT surgeons' operations are on private patients, with huge variations existing between individual surgeons.

Inequalities of waiting times

No large scale comparison of ENT waiting times in the NHS and the private sector has been undertaken. However, NHS waiting times for an out-patient appointment averaged over 14 weeks in 1994 and, in some cases, were over 1 year. The few enquiries made to private rooms always resulted in the offer of an appointment within 3 weeks.

In summary, we have a specialty in which the surgeons are only given 2 or 3 NHS operating lists per week. This alone goes a long way to explaining very low levels of surgical workload on the part of some of its consultants. However, we should ask why the NHS does not offer the specialty more operating capacity before considering further consultant appointments. Furthermore, the specialty has an enormous amount of discretion in deciding whether or not an operation is needed. In such circumstances it may be unwise to allow individuals the opportunity to increase their income by simply varying criteria which have inadequate scientific verification. An ENT surgeon told me that when he was at medical school his professor said, 'It is a poor ENT surgeon who looks down a throat and cannot see 25 guineas.' Today's value is more likely to be £500.

THE OPHTHALMOLOGY JIGSAW

Ophthalmology is a specialty that deals virtually exclusively with the eye, and no other specialty overlaps it to any significant extent. Unlike most other specialties, it is set against a cultural background in which the population is used to paying for the care of its eyes. The nation has accepted the need for many of its citizens to pay for spectacles and, in recent years, has had to get used to paying for eye tests.

Ophthalmology is predominantly an out-patient specialty with most of its patients attending clinics and day-case suites for medical and laser treatments, rather than being admitted to a hospital bed. Most of an ophthalmologist's working week is therefore concerned with treatments in those locations, rather than in the operating theatre.

Surgical discretion

The most common operations for this specialty are those involving cataract surgery, which represents over half of the operative workload. The operation is considered highly effective and appropriate, although there is dispute over the precise point at which surgical intervention is desirable. The second most common operation is for the correction of squint. Whilst it could be argued that there is some cosmetic element to this procedure, in the main, the specialty does not have the wide level of discretion that is seen in some other specialties.

Contractual issues

Ophthalmologists usually have 2 operating lists per week and 4 or 5 out-patient clinics. If the 2 operating lists are shared with junior staff, a consultant may be restricted to only 3 hours operating per week. This specialty does not have a high volume of on call commitment and operations outside working hours are unusual for a consultant.

A consultant may be allocated up to 5 clinics per week, but not all ophthalmologists do this number. Uncommitted sessions are not checked by managers and, in some locations, allegations of contractual abuse have not been addressed by managers. Health authorities allow for travelling times between home and hospital within the working week and allow a reduction in contractual time for travel between nearby hospitals. In one hospital a consultant team operated on 538 cases in 1 year, but the consultant personally operated on only 178 of those patients. Of those, 96 were private patients, all operated on in his NHS sessions. This situation continued unchecked by NHS managers and even when it was brought to their attention they took no action. Years later, after that surgeon had retired, his successor still uses a third of his theatre sessions to operate on private patients.

NHS volume

The average ophthalmology team operates on 10–11 patients per week, and if we assume half of that work is done by juniors, the average ophthalmologist does 5 operations per week in the NHS. Indeed, many do less than 3 per week. In the sample of ophthalmologists studied, very few attended the 5 out-patient sessions recommended by their College. Ophthalmologists see an average of 33 new out-patients per week in a 46-week year, which would mean 6 or 7 new patients in each of 5 clinics per week. In practice there is a tendency to have 2 very busy main clinics, with the specialist clinics attended by small numbers of patients.

Private sector operating

In 1992–93 it is estimated that 16 000 cataract and 10 000 other ophthalmology operations were performed in independent hospitals in England and Wales. This represents an average of only 1 private operation per consultant per week.

Rooms commitments

A sample of 70 consultants showed a very high level of attendance in private rooms sessions during the normal working week. Committing 2, 3 or even 4 sessions per week to private rooms must make it difficult to fulfil contractual obligations to the NHS.

Balance of surgery

In terms of operations, this specialty appears to have about 1 private operation to 5 NHS operations undertaken by consultants. The problem of the balance between NHS and private sector out-patient activity is much more difficult to assess.

Inequalities of waiting times

NHS patients wait for an average of over 19 weeks with some patients waiting over 1 year for an appointment, whereas the wait to see an ophthalmic surgeon is only 2–3 weeks in the private sector. This situation has existed for over 20 years in some towns and cities.

In summary, the specialty faces growing demand as the average age of the population increases and yet surgeons are only offered 2 operating sessions per week. In many cases these have to be shared with trainee surgeons and some of our most skilful surgeons are left operating for fewer than 3 hours per week. There is a heavy demand for out-patient clinics and yet ophthalmologists on maximum part-time NHS contracts can routinely be found consulting in the private sector for 2, 3 and even 4 half-days during the normal working week.

THE TRAUMA AND ORTHOPAEDIC JIGSAW

The title of 'trauma and orthopaedics' reflects the dual nature of this specialty. In simple terms, the trauma side deals with accidents and emergencies (particularly broken bones). The orthopaedic side is concerned with the treatment of diseases, such as arthritis, which often requires planned surgical admission. Much of the emergency work is handled by junior surgeons who will call in consultants for help with difficult cases.

Surgical discretion

About half of this specialty's operative workload is concerned with emergency work, where there is certainly less scope for discretion about whether or not a patient actually needs an operation. Most of the discretion in this specialty relates to the best time to intervene and which of the 37 types of replacement joint to use. The failure to adequately assess which joint replacement models are most and least successful has led to criticism that as many as 1 in 5 hip operations are now revisions of previously failed operations (Jones 1995). Not all of these are due to mechanical failure, but the differing levels of success are sufficient to worry many surgeons – and should worry even more patients. There also appears to be a backlog in demand for some types of joint replacement surgery from the large and growing elderly population that has still to benefit from this technique.

Contractual issues

Most consultants in this specialty have 3 operating lists and 3 out-patient clinics per week. The type and level of commitment that consultants display is heavily dependent on the level of junior staff support available. In some well staffed hospitals consultant orthopaedic surgeons devote virtually all of their time to planned rather than emergency surgery. Contractual problems can be encountered when the high level of junior support available enables consultants to leave much of the emergency work to those juniors.

NHS volume

The survey of 120 consultants represents a large sample of the specialty's senior surgeons. For that sample to show, as it does, an average of only 4–5 NHS operations per consultant per week (and to reveal that a fifth of consultants did 3 or fewer operations per week) raises serious doubts about the way the NHS runs its orthopaedic service. It must be remembered that, except in the smaller and isolated hospitals where consultants have limited junior support, most emergency operating is done by juniors. It is rare to see consultants doing emergency operations at weekends or at night. The NHS needs to reflect on whether or not it is reasonable to allow so little planned operating to be undertaken without any compensating emergency commitment.

Private sector operating

In 1992, the 832 trauma and orthopaedic surgeons in England and Wales undertook over 71 000 operations in independent hospitals. For a 46-week year that produces an average of just under 2 private operations per week.

Rooms commitments

The study of 177 orthopaedic surgeons revealed that almost 90% spent at least 1 half-day per week in their rooms and that half of the consultants spent 2 or more half-days each working week on private consultations.

Balance of surgery

Over 5 years ago more than 1 hip replacement in 4 was undertaken on private patients and the proportion is now even higher.

BUPA claim that 30% of all hip replacements are now done in the private sector. For some consultants, up to half of their operating is said to be on private patients and some junior surgeons embark on their careers with the attitude that the NHS is a form of 'loss-leader' which gives them a foot in the door to a lucrative association with the private sector. When discussing how to reduce the large NHS orthopaedic waiting list in one town, we were advised by one surgeon to consider using the private sector, 'because I personally do more hip operations there than in the Health Service'. This surgeon held a maximum part-time contract which obliged him to 'devote substantially the whole of his time to the NHS'.

Inequalities of waiting times

Waiting times for an out-patient appointment in the NHS have consistently been amongst the worst in the country. An average wait of over 25 weeks, with many people waiting over 1 year, just to see a surgeon is one of the very worst features of British life. The alternative is to reach for a wallet in order to be seen by the same surgeon in just 2 or 3 weeks.

In summary, the average orthopaedic surgeon performed less than 5 operations in NHS hospitals and 2 in independent hospitals each working week. Each had 3 NHS clinics per week and over half of them had 2 or more private rooms sessions per week.

THE HEART OF THE MATTER?

The evidence presented in this book does not conclusively link the way the surgical profession works in the private sector with the inequality of waiting time experienced by patients. One key piece of evidence is always missing – that of how much operating each individual surgeon does in the private sector. Table 6.2 summarizes the evidence presented for the three specialties examined above and highlights the gap in the information about what surgeons do in the private sector in relation to their NHS commitments. It is that link which is at the heart of the investigators' problem. Strangely, it was matters of the heart that gave me the strongest clue yet about a link between inequality and working for two masters.

Table 6.2   Linking systems failure to inequitable access

Subject matter	ENT	Supporting evidence in Ophthalmology	Orthopaedics
1. Surgical discretion	✓✓	✓	✓
2. Contractual issues	✓	✓	✓
3. Low NHS volume	✓	✓	✓
4. High private sector operating	?	?	?
5. Regular rooms commitments	?	✓✓	✓✓
6. Disproportionate balance of surgery	?	?	✓
7 Inequality of waiting times	✓	✓✓	✓✓

Key:
✓✓ = Strong supporting evidence
✓ = Some supporting evidence
? = Not much evidence available

A long wait for any operation can be frustrating, inconvenient and painful, but in some extreme cases, too long a wait might mean death. The media headlines which describe 'death on a waiting list' most commonly relate to one particular surgical specialty – cardiac surgery. Cardiac surgeons specialize in heart operations and 80–90% of cardiac operations are undertaken to try and alleviate the problems caused by coronary heart disease. If the arteries supplying blood to the heart muscle become choked it causes pain (which we call angina), or even death of part of the muscle (which we know as a heart attack or myocardial infarction).

Coronary heart disease is more common in certain groups of people than others. In particular, it is more common amongst the elderly, people of South Asian origin, those living in areas of socio-economic deprivation and those who are heavy smokers, have poor dietary patterns and undertake limited physical activity. Very many people have the disease without having any recognizable symptoms, but it is estimated that between 11% and 17% of those over the age of 65 have angina, a figure that increases to 22% for those over the age of 70. Cardiac disease is the cause of death for almost 30% of the British population and is by far the most common cause of death.

Whilst the death rate is highest amongst the elderly, the effect of this condition on the middle-aged is also severe. In 1987 it was calculated that coronary heart disease was the cause of 25% of all years of working life lost for men under 65 and 15% of years of working life lost for women (London Implementation Group 1993). The United Kingdom has one of the worst mortality rates for cardiac disease in the world and has failed to achieve the marked reductions seen in the USA, Canada, Australia and some European countries.

When prevention has failed and medical treatment is no longer likely to succeed, then a coronary artery bypass graft (CABG) is seen as the surgical solution. This operation involves taking veins from elsewhere in the patient's body to replace the diseased arteries. The veins are usually taken from the leg or arm. The actual operation takes about 2 hours, but the patient will be in the operating theatre for $2^1/_2$–3 hours to enable all the preparatory work and follow-up checks to take place. These operations are truly a matter of life or death. In Britain, our cardiac surgeons perform about 17 000 CABG operations per year. This meets the government's target that the NHS should achieve 300 operations per million population, but the British Cardiac Society believe the rate should be double that to meet the needs of the population.

In 1992, a major review of surgical services in the London area was established and one of the specialties involved was cardiac surgery (London Implementation Group 1993). A multi-disciplinary group was given the task of establishing how many cardiac units were needed in London and to ascertain whether or not there was any scope for rationalization. The group discovered that 14 NHS hospitals had cardiac units employing 39 cardiac surgeons, who collectively undertook 6763 CABGs on adults in 1992. The data they gathered identified what work was done in each NHS hospital, but did not identify which surgeons undertook the operations.

Along with a group of colleagues, I was commissioned to examine the theatre registers of the 14 NHS hospitals in London that undertook cardiac surgery. We obtained photostat copies of the registers for the months of September, October and November 1992. The study involved over 30 theatre registers. Each register presented information in a different fashion. Some did not record operating times, and two did not record the individual surgeon who undertook the operation. Despite the difficulties, two detailed studies were possible. The first covered all the hospitals and simply gathered the numbers of operations undertaken by each consultant, except for 2 hospitals where the number of operations could only be gathered for each team. A second, more detailed, study covered 9 hospitals for the 3-month period and looked at information such as the start and finish time of each operation, the type of operation performed, the name of the surgeon and assistant and the age of the patient.

By complete coincidence, this study was taking place at the same time as Professor Brian Williams of Sheffield University was undertaking a study of the workload of all independent hospitals in England and Wales. Both groups were bound by confidentiality agreements that meant we could not divulge information about individual surgeons or hospitals. We were, however, able to compare information on a regional basis. At that time, England had 14 health regions. It was therefore possible to compare Williams' study of cardiac surgery done in the independent hospitals within the four Thames regions with the work I had undertaken in the 14 London hospitals, which were the only NHS hospitals in those same regions. Whilst I could not get a perfect picture of what each individual surgeon did, I could look at the collective efforts of the 39 surgeons in the two sectors.

In 1992, 6763 CABGs were conducted in the 14 NHS London hospitals. Some of these were performed on private patients, but the theatre registers do not consistently record the paying status of patients and strangely there is no requirement for them to do so. Nevertheless, over the 3-month study period we identified 39 private patients which, given the fact that some registers were not recording private patients, suggests a minimum of 160 private patients per year. I believe the figure is more likely to be in excess of 350, given the pressure in some units to increase the earnings in NHS private wings. Over the same 3-month period we examined the division of work between the various grades and types of surgeon in 9 of the 14 hospitals involved. This revealed that 46% of the operations were performed by NHS consultants, 21% by academic staff of consultant status and 32% by juniors in training.

In the same year, Williams (personal communication 1994b) estimated that in the private sector there were 4025 CABGs in the four Thames' regions, although only 1545 were known to be on patients residing in England and Wales. The remaining patients were predominantly from Eire and Europe, with a small number from elsewhere in the world. We do not actually know who did these operations, but with the help of a general practitioner, and as a result of telephone enquiries, I obtained a list of the cardiac surgeons working in each of the independent hospitals. Virtually all the staff listed were NHS consultants, and many worked in two or three private hospitals. One consultant was on the lists of four such hospitals. The hospitals also listed one surgeon who no longer operates in the NHS, although he has an honorary NHS contract. We were not given the names of surgeons who had retired, surgeons holding academic appointments, surgeons from elsewhere in England or of visiting surgeons from overseas. This does not mean that such surgeons do not operate privately in these independent hospitals, but it seems reasonable to assume that few CABG operations are conducted by such surgeons. We must therefore conclude that most of the 4025 operations were conducted by NHS consultants.

A summary of the results of these two studies appears in Table 6.3. In simplified terms, the situation in London in 1992 was:

- 37% of CABGs took place in non-NHS hospitals
- 40% of CABGs were performed on private patients
- 50% of the operations performed by NHS consultant and academic staff were on private patients
- 60% of the operations performed by NHS consultants were on private patients.

Some will argue that this grossly over-estimates the amount of private surgery undertaken by NHS surgeons, but others say it is an under-estimate as far as some individual surgeons are

Table 6.3 Estimate of coronary artery bypass operations in London in 1992

Of 10 788 coronary artery bypass operations performed 6763 were in NHS hospitals

Of 10 788 CABGs at least 4185, possibly in excess of 4375, were performed on private patients

About 2164 NHS operations were performed by junior staff, whereas most of the 4185–4375 private patients were operated on by consultant and academic surgeons

NHS surgeons performed about 7204 operations. About 2761 to 2951 were NHS and they probably did most of 4185 to 4375 private operations concerned. When the London study was in progress, one of the cardiac study group was discussing the NHS–private balance with a surgeon who claimed that in 1 year he did 100 operations in the NHS and 400 in the private sector. I can confirm that he did only 100 in the NHS, but even though I know which private hospitals he works in, and how frequently he visits those hospitals, I cannot be sure exactly how many private operations he performed in the independent hospitals. No-one other than the surgeon himself knows that – so he is either prone to gross exaggeration or he does indeed do 80% of his operating on private patients, despite holding a maximum part-time NHS contract.

The work I did was commissioned by the London Implementation Group (LIG) committee but was never published. During the course of the project I was surprised, and worried, by the low level of NHS activity we discovered. I shared my findings with a retired cardiac surgeon who had been a professional colleague for over 20 years. He had spent all of his career with access to only one theatre, but yet had routinely done six major operations each week. He scanned down the list of each consultant's operative workload until he reached the figure of 1.2 operations per week. He could scarcely contain his anger as he enquired, 'What is this – a **** hobby?'

When the final report was completed I was asked to deliver two copies, by hand, to London and to return the copies of the theatre registers I had been working on. No-one was available to discuss the findings on the day I delivered the report, but on the following day I received a telephone call requesting that I withdraw two pages at the end of the report. I was told that my comments on private practice were too strong. At one point it was thought that the report might go forward under my signature to the Chairman of LIG or perhaps go forward under the specialty chairman's signature with sections of my report replaced with 'some weaselly words'.

In the event, sections of the report were deleted and I was told it was later discussed with the Secretary of State and Sir Duncan Nichol. It was thought that there were enough politically difficult decisions to be taken about the possible closure of some cardiac units – why add to them by drawing attention to a potential link between low workload in the NHS and activity in the private sector? The cardiac review team members were not even shown the report, nor were the findings discussed with the cardiac surgeons concerned. Despite the initial enthusiasm which met our early findings (in a reference to our work, it was said that the panel had put the right ferret up the right hole), the final report was shortened and its findings hidden. The fact is, there is a lot to hide.

INCOMPLETE PICTURES

Doubtless to the relief of many, the confidentiality of some data, the complete absence of data in some areas and the difficulty of linking data from different sources, inevitably results in an incomplete picture. No-one in this country can produce a substantial survey of large groups of surgeons identifying precisely what each one does in the NHS and in the private sector, and how that relates to waiting time for their patients. The jigsaw is incomplete. However, even though the few missing pieces mean an irritating absence of some detail, the overall picture is clear.

Those who cannot afford to pay for treatment wait longer to get their treatment, get treated less frequently, are less likely to be operated on by a consultant and suffer greater levels of illness. The insured and the wealthy get treated more quickly, have more than their fair share of operations, are more likely to be operated on by a consultant and are likely to have lower levels of illness. The latter group, however, is not without its problems. They pay extra money unnecessarily to jump false queues and undergo more than their fair share of unnecessary surgery.

Winston Churchill said that to understand the future we need to understand the past. He argued that the NHS should be like the fire brigade of his day, which went to both the humble cottage and rich man's mansion. Instead, we have a health care system which is more like the fire brigade of earlier times. Over a century ago you could find signs on some houses and barns indicating that the building was covered by an insurance company. If the house was on fire the private fire brigade of the time would know whether or not they need put the fire out. If the sign belonged to a company by whom they were retained they would take action; if not, they would pass by. We are now returning to a health care system beset by the very inequality the NHS was designed to remove. One-tenth of our patients received one-fifth of the planned operations that our surgeons undertake and a small, but increasing, proportion of our surgeons are now carrying out more than half their work in the private sector.

A tale of two cities?

The inequality of health care between the two cities is not always clear, because the two cities are some distance apart. The citizens of the first city enjoy living there; their numbers include the politicians, civil servants and managers who run the two systems and the surgeons who work in both systems. The citizens of the second city are left with no clear insight into just how different the standards are between the two cities.

7

TIME FOR CHANGE?

THE NEED FOR CHANGE

This book has examined whether or not patients and the NHS itself suffer as a result of the way private medicine is conducted in Britain; its conclusion is that they do. We find surgeons are allowed to work for two competing employers in a way not permitted in commercial practice, nor in public life. There is neither an adequate consultant contract nor a monitoring mechanism in place to identify any abuse. The NHS does not know where its key employees are during the working day, nor has it any idea of the actual amount of work undertaken by any individual surgeon. Surgeons have too much scope to neglect the NHS in favour of their private work and at the same time we find hugely different waiting times to see the same surgeon in the two competing sectors.

The National Health Service has a statutory requirement to ensure that private practice does not, to a significant extent, interfere with the performance of the NHS, or disadvantage non-paying patients. The Department of Health acknowledges this statutory requirement and claims it was the main principle agreed with the medical profession when determining the conduct of private practice in National Health Service hospitals. It argues that this requirement is best met by local managers having a firm grip on what their consultants do and that this can be achieved through the use of job plans. It is, however, quite clear that no such controls are in operation. Audit Commission and National Audit Office studies have discovered that in many cases job plans are not available, or that when they are, they are out of date. The flexible nature of the consultants' contract is such that managers have no clear guidance about how much time consultants should be allowed to spend in the private sector. The only serious attempt to define this, made by Sir Duncan Nichol, was subsequently undermined by civil servants and politicians.

The inequality and inefficiency in the British health care system is unacceptable. In January 1995, I presented some preliminary evidence in advance of this book, in a television documentary and accompanying booklet entitled *Serving two masters* (Yates 1995a, Yates 1995b). At that time I argued that three steps needed to be taken simultaneously.

1. The gathering of detailed evidence about the actual work done by surgeons in the NHS and in the private sector.
2. The production of clear guidance about the contractual obligations of consultants working in the NHS.
3. An explanation of why ministers, Department of Health officials, NHS managers and auditors have been so reluctant to address this issue.

Reaction to the television programme was a mixture of enthusiastic support, apathy and rejection. Over 100 letters and telephone calls were received in the first 2 weeks following transmission, a response the director had never before seen in his long career of television documentary production. The vast majority of letters came from patients, all over Britain, giving examples of queue jumping and problems in securing outpatient appointments or hospital admission. Some people wrote simply to express thanks that the issue had been raised. The letters included these stories and others like them.

- A Hertfordshire patient who had already waited over a year to see an ophthalmologist was told by the surgeon, 'if I paid for a private consultation it would only be a matter of days before I could see him and that I could still opt for NHS treatment and probably get treated quicker as a result'.
- A lady from Devon said, 'The surgeon who did my hip operation privately and who also saw me privately at his rooms for many years lost interest when I said I could not afford another private operation and I was then put on to another man.'
- After three heart attacks a man from Preston asked to be referred by his GP to a cardiologist. He was told by the consultant, 'that he did not think he could even get me on a waiting list and even if he could I may wait *years* before I was seen'. The patient went privately and was seen in days.
- An almost identical story from Suffolk, but the patient chose not to go privately and after 7 months was still waiting for a hospital appointment.
- In January 1994, a Derbyshire man saw a cardiac surgeon who told him he needed a major operation. It was said that it would be 6 months to a year before he would be called. A year later a letter offering him a bed arrived on the very day the Channel 4 programme was screened. His wife had to tell the hospital that he had died 7 months previously.

I also had letters from NHS staff, including theatre sisters, porters, mortuary technicians, physiotherapists, occupational therapists, general practitioners, anaesthetists, surgeons and health authority chairmen. They related their own experiences of dubious practice, and even fraud. One consultant told me that 'many have become disillusioned with the NHS and are turning to private medicine'. A surgeon talking about the careers of his colleagues said, 'The prospect of substantial financial gain however, if not dominant at the outset, soon becomes the main motivation.'

In the House of Commons, Early Day Motion No. 415 1995 was put to the House on the day the report was published. It said:

This House calls on the Secretary of State for Health to investigate urgently the report by John Yates, the Government's own waiting list advisor, that NHS surgeons are spending NHS time on private patients; and further calls on her to investigate vigorous monitoring of consultants' time to ensure that their principal obligations to the NHS are honoured.

It was signed by 104 Labour MPs, but only one Liberal and one Conservative MP. On 25 January Mrs Margaret Beckett, the Opposition Spokesman for Health Care, placed a written question (Beckett 1995), 'To ask the Secretary of State for Health, if she will undertake an enquiry to establish the extent to which NHS consultants are not fulfilling their NHS contracts.' The next day, the junior minister, Mr Malone replied, 'No. National Health Service employers are responsible for ensuring that individual NHS consultants are fulfilling their contractual obligations.'

The response of the Government was consistent with the desire to disentangle the centre from any responsibility for day-to-day management of the Health Service, although it was disappointing to see that Mrs Bottomley, who had previously been so keen to champion the need to examine consultants' contracts, was now rejecting a call for such an examination. It was, however, helpful to have an explicit statement that the responsibility lay with NHS employing authorities. Whilst those authorities lack any national guidance, the disinterest of the government does, at least, mean that individual employing authorities will now have to clarify contractual uncertainties themselves.

The response from the professionals in the NHS was decidedly low key. One senior NHS manager told me there was nothing in the programme or the report that was not already known to all managers and clinicians in the NHS. The Hospital Consultants and Specialists Association and the British Medical Association reiterated their views on the interpretation of the consultants' contract. Both maintained that consultants could, indeed, spend up to 2 whole days per week working in the private sector, despite their holding maximum part-time NHS contracts. They argued that the onerous responsibilities of a consultant surgeon in the NHS with regard to research, teaching, audit, administration, ward rounds and other tasks, can be undertaken in the evenings and at weekends in order to allow those same surgeons to work in the private sector for up to 2 whole days during the working week.

The most questionable attack came from a BMA spokesman, who accused me of having a far left-wing tendency. What he and some of the extreme right-wing politicians should understand is that many of those who deeply resent the inequalities in our society are Conservative voters. Concern about equality is not a left-wing ideology. In my case, it is part of a Christian ethic, but concern for equality is not restricted to Christianity nor any other form of theology. What should concern us is that there are too many people on the far right wing of politics, and in the BMA, who seem to have no regard for equality. They should be cautious in classifying those who want to see a change for the better as either left wing, controversial or unreasonable.

George Bernard Shaw said, 'The reasonable man adapts himself to the world; the unreasonable one persists in trying to adapt the world to himself. Therefore all progress depends on the unreasonable man.' I have been heartened to see signs of unreasonable men emerging in the NHS. When the new Chief Executive of the NHS, Mr Alan Langlands, was asked whether his predecessor's comments about limiting consultants private sessions were still in force he replied, 'A good question,' and went on to say that the claims that consultants are devoting much more time to private practice than guidance allows 'cannot be disregarded' (Langlands 1995). The President of The Institute of Health Services Management, Peter Stansby, said on the Channel 4 programme (Yates 1995a), 'We as managers have to do something about it.' Dr Jeremy Lee-Potter, former Chairman of the British Medical Association Council, acknowledged that there was public disquiet about doctors 'moonlighting' in the private sector, and called for a new consultant contract (Laurance 1995): 'We need to re-negotiate a clean straightforward contract which makes it clearer where consultants are expected to be and when.' A review of the television programme in the *British Medical Journal* was entitled 'Embarrassing greed' (Bulstrode 1995a) and the author was 'left deeply embarrassed that I belong to a profession which has shown itself both unwilling and unable to set standards that would make this documentary unnecessary'. A senior member of the Royal College of Surgeons wrote to me (personal communication 1995) saying, 'I must admit to being somewhat shocked and surprised by any suggestion that more than two [half-days] were used by 10/11 session consultants.' That surgeon is not alone in believing that a full investigation is needed.

Despite this support, my call for an enquiry has so far been ignored. Politicians, NHS managers and surgeons themselves have not been prepared to take up the challenge to undertake a systematic review of the workload of consultant surgeons in the NHS and the private sector. The Audit Commission (1995) revealed (2 months after my report was published) that there was evidence that the surgeons who did a large volume of private practice tended to be those who did a low volume of NHS work. Despite the fact that their evidence matches my findings, we still find no willingness to investigate if workload is adequate and whether it is fairly distributed. Just in case there should be a change of heart, the Appendix to this book outlines the case for a two-pronged enquiry. I do not call for such an enquiry to establish whether or not there is a problem, but to establish the magnitude of the problem that without doubt exists.

Regrettably, it looks as if those of us who want to achieve change will now have to move towards solutions without an adequate knowledge base. This is not the ideal way to proceed – it was a knee-jerk reaction to cash crises and waiting list problems, rather than a thorough examination of the facts, that led to the latest reforms of the NHS. This was succinctly described by Sir Raymond Hoffenberg (1994), 'instead of "get ready, taken aim, fire" the government chose "get ready, fire, take aim" '. However, given the secrecy surrounding the work of surgeons in the NHS and the private sector it seems we must now consider solutions without the benefit of an enquiry.

OPTIONS FOR CHANGE

For those who wish to introduce more equality of access to health care, there are several options that can be considered. Some would involve fundamental changes to the health care system; others can be classed as minor modifications to the existing basic structure. Radical solutions could range from the total abolition of private health care to the complete privatization of the whole system. Between those two extremes lie the four intermediate options discussed below.

Complete separation of NHS and private medicine

In such a system there would be no private patient work permitted in the NHS and no NHS surgeons would be permitted to do private practice outside the Service. There are strong grounds, according to conventional business ethics, public organization probity and the moral ethic, to suggest that there is no place for surgeons who work in both sectors. If NHS surgeons were paid a higher salary and not allowed to undertake any private work then the current unethical system of working for two employers would cease and the NHS and the private sector could compete on an equal footing for work.

All private work to be conducted in NHS institutions

Another solution would be to ensure that all private care takes place in NHS hospitals. It would be up to the purchasing authority, or some external agent, to monitor the level of service provided by hospitals and surgeons, to ensure that gross inequalities of access do not occur. This option would allow the population to exercise some choice as to whether they pay privately for health care or rely on state provision.

All surgeons to leave the NHS and become private contractors

If the NHS did not directly employ any surgeons at all (in the same way that it does not employ general practitioners) it could simply contract with competing surgeons to undertake work. All surgeons would be self-employed, working in a similar fashion to the legal profession, and would therefore be subject to market forces.

Move to an insurance-based system

The British health care system is unusual in that virtually all services provided by private hospitals are to patients whose choice has been to insure or pay cash for private operations. The introduction of compulsory health care insurance for those who could afford it, with the state paying for the insurance of those who could not, would enable private hospitals to take patients from either group. The same would apply to NHS hospitals. The NHS and the private sector could co-exist and compete, providing there was some mechanism for protecting the needs of consumers as individuals, and ensuring that the NHS and the taxpayer were not disadvantaged by such a system.

The trouble with the sort of major re-organizations suggested above is that whilst they are directed at achieving changes in patient care, they rarely do so. The professionals become so busy defending their own position that they do not focus their attention on the issues of improving the access to care for patients. This means that whichever direction future governments choose to travel, we need to establish mechanisms that force politicians, managers and the medical profession to give fair access to care for all patients.

CHANGE IS COMING ANYWAY?

My concern in this book is equality of access to hospital care for all patients regardless of their ability to pay. If, in the near future, the National Health Service makes considerable strides in shortening waiting times for both in-patient admission and out-patient appointments, my concerns about inequality would be ill-founded. Some senior NHS managers are already talking about the establishment of waiting-free zones; if they are successful in achieving this, and can widen these zones to include the whole of Britain, patients will be able to relax in the knowledge that they will receive speedy health care when it is needed. These optimists argue that my analysis of the experience of patients over the past decade and the identification of inequalities is outdated. They contend that in the near future the NHS will radically reduce waiting time for all members of society and we will then be thankful that a new and more efficient NHS will have succeeded for the first time since 1948 in meeting its objective of equal access to health care for all British citizens. However, the politicians and managers who support this view are playing for high stakes. Once again, we may find ourselves trying to achieve radical reductions in waiting time in the highly charged atmosphere of the run-up to a general election.

My analysis is more pessimistic. I believe that long waiting times are caused by a lethal cocktail of underprovision of resources and inefficiency in the use of those resources. I also believe that the long waiting times experienced by the poorer members of our society are caused in part by the way in which the NHS and the private sector interface. If the NHS fails to deliver equal access in the near future, I contend that politicians, surgeons and managers will be forced to review the contractual position of consultant surgeons and the work they undertake. Eventually, patients, and society as a whole, will demand change. Will those groups in a position to act take up the challenge to negotiate a reasonable change now, or will patient power have to force them to change later?

NEGOTIATING A MEANINGFUL AND LASTING CHANGE

Achieving equality and efficiency in hospital care is a complex problem. A strategy which will achieve fundamental and long-lasting change will need the cooperation of politicians, surgeons, managers and the public and it will involve a complex grouping of actions. It will not be sufficient to simply agree a new contract; it must be placed in a setting which will allow it to bear fruit. The conditions for success will include most or all of the six features discussed below.

Establish an evidence-based independent inspectorate

The past few years have seen the introduction of an improved research strategy in the NHS. There has been much emphasis placed on obtaining accurate evidence about the appropriateness and cost effectiveness of interventions. To date, this excellent strategy has been passive; it now needs to progress to being interventive. Simply gathering research findings together is not sufficient – there needs to be a further step which examines existing practice to see how well it conforms to those findings.

All surgical workload must be monitored by a research based independent inspectorate, regardless of whether the individual surgeon's activity takes place in the NHS, the private sector or both. All surgery needs to be assessed against the background of contemporary scientific evidence. The work of an independent inspectorate should include the identification of situations where surgical intervention is:

- inappropriate (should not be offered at all or in such a quantity to a given population)
- insufficient (too little treatment for a given population)
- dangerous (e.g. undertaken by a surgeon with insufficient experience or one who is an 'occasional' surgeon)
- inefficient (e.g. using an inappropriate level of resources).

Determine the surgical needs of the population

Evidence-based research should be used to establish reasonable parameters for referral rates, admission rates and operation rates for each specialty and for the more common conditions and operative procedures. We need to establish whether the three- to fivefold variation that we commonly find in surgical activity in similar populations can be justified. This will require investigative studies on both extremes of all rates and, given changes over time, will need continuous updating.

Determine the patients' requirements

Patients and their relatives must be involved in setting standards regarding minimum waiting times for both out-patient appointments and operative procedures. The process has already commenced with the establishment of Charter standards (Department of Health 1995), but may well require greater patient, rather than politician, involvement. The process can most easily start with waiting times, but may well progress into other areas where the patient's perception of quality can be reasonably measured. I would be surprised if patients would accept that any out-patient waiting times should normally be in excess of 1 month, or that waiting time for an in-patient admission should exceed 3 months.

Establish minimum provision levels and recommended workload levels

Having established the likely needs of a population, we must then identify an agreed minimum level of resource support to enable those needs to be met. This will require the determination of the appropriate level of surgeons, support staff, beds, theatre sessions and other resources.

It will not be sufficient to merely establish minimum levels of resource provision; this must be done in conjunction with the establishment of reasonable consultant workload standards. To date, managers and surgeons have no agreements at all about surgical workload. Negotiated agreements specifying the range of activity that can be reasonably expected would be helpful for both managers and surgeons. Once resource levels and workload standards were agreed, a surgeon could not be unfairly criticized for working at a low level if he did not have the minimum resources specified. The negotiations about workload agreements would have to take account of who undertakes the operation, the surgeon or his junior, and also take account of non-operative activity undertaken, particularly in relation to teaching, administration etc. The current amount of operating undertaken by surgeons is considerably lower than the public might reasonably expect. This solution will either require more funds for the NHS, a reduction in the number of surgeons employed, or a radical examination of activity to identify and eradicate unnecessary surgery.

Produce nationally agreed consultants' contracts

A nationally agreed contract framework should specify responsibilities to be covered, hours to be worked and the workload that can be expected. NHS contracts should ensure that there are at least eight fixed sessions for operating and clinics in a working week, during normal working hours. If any reduction in the eight clinical sessions per week was negotiated to take account of on call commitments, then all time spent in hospital during on call periods must be logged, or other convincing evidence produced to support the loss of fixed sessions.

Evening working might be appropriate in some circumstances, although one would not expect surgeons to be operating routinely in the morning, afternoon and evening of the same day. It might, for instance, be appropriate to arrange for evening clinics when a surgeon is on call for that evening and night if one, or both, of the morning and afternoon sessions immediately prior to that had been devoted to research or audit, rather than operating or out-patient clinics.

Control of private practice activity

Where private practice is permitted it should be subject to control by the independent inspectorate. Two models of organizing a mixture of NHS and private sector activity could be considered.

1. Complete separation where surgeons work either for the NHS or the private sector, but not both.
2. NHS surgeons are permitted to work in the private sector during evenings and weekends, but not during the working day.

If there is a complete separation of the two sectors then NHS surgeons will have to be paid more money to work in the NHS. One of the reasons why private practice is undertaken by so many surgeons is quite simply that it is a very easy way of doubling their incomes. For many surgeons there would be little incentive to even consider private practice if the NHS made a more reasonable financial offer for their services. Compared with salaries in the City and some sections of industry and commerce, surgeons are not well paid. As a percentage of total public expenditure, doubling the salary of all consultant surgeons would not involve huge sums of money; however, it would leave the NHS in some difficulty in relation to the remaining 15000 consultants in other specialties.

If the model of permitting NHS surgeons to undertake private practice outside normal working hours is adopted, then certain control mechanisms will need to be considered. For such surgeons no private practice should be permitted if:

- agreed workload standards (both in terms of the number of operations and new out-patients) had not been met

or

- there was evidence of under-access in terms of referral, admission or operation rate or excessive waiting time in relation to the standards set unless the independent inspectorate had agreed that the under-access rates or the long waiting time were due to factors outside the surgeon's control (e.g. the health authorities and hospitals were not providing sufficient resources).

FORCING CHANGE

It is often considered unfair to name surgeons and managers for apparent failures in health care when they are clearly just small pawns in a huge game. It is argued that it is the system that is failing and thus the individual should not take the blame. But however unpalatable it may be, the fact is that tackling systems will mean tackling people. Each of us shoulders some responsibility for the inequitable situation that we find ourselves in. It is our responsibility to put things right for the benefit of the patients we are serving. The fact that those either side of us fail to react, does not justify our own inaction. We need to seek allies amongst consumer groups, managers, trades unions, politicians, clinicians and the church. These allies need to work together, but they will require the help of change agents and leaders who can sustain a campaign over a period of time.

If long waiting times for the poorer sections of our society remain, and if politicians, surgeons and managers continue to be apathetic, there are a number of steps, discussed below, that can be taken.

Establish an aggressive consumer protection system

Despite the best efforts of the Consumers' Association, the Patients' Association, Community Health Councils and the College of Health, patients still experience unacceptably long waits for treatment. Greater pressure could be exerted by establishing a single issue pressure group, solely devoted to studying waiting times in both the NHS and the private sector, for both in-patient admission and out-patient appointment. This 'wait watchers' organization would need to publish data, act as a general watchdog, and act on behalf of individual patients to put pressure on hospitals and surgeons to treat patients more speedily. It would advertise its services in local newspapers and on the television, and in the event of total apathy on the part of the government, management and the medical profession, may even resort to a 'suburban guerrilla' style of picketing on behalf of those suffering from the extremes of inequality.

Establish a series of debates on the ethical issues of paying for health care

There are many groups in society who share concern about the inequitable system that faces many patients today. Currently these groups are rather isolated and there may be merit in coordinating a collective searching of the conscience by politicians from all parties, clinicians, church leaders, trades union representatives and National Health Service managers. A programme of debates should be established, the purpose of which would be to try to modify the practice of surgeons, managers and patients by examining publicly some of the following issues:

1. How is it that doctors can let cash decide clinical priorities?
2. Is it reasonable for patients to pay cash in order to jump the queue?
3. How can patients be sure that the NHS is working efficiently?
4. How can patients be sure that they are not paying twice when they decide to go privately?
5. What methods can society use to expose the unfairness of the current situation?

Exert commercial pressure

A large proportion of private insurance premiums are paid for by employers. Many are concerned about the high level of expenditure they are incurring on behalf of their employees. Some employers are already beginning to question whether this 'perk' is as beneficial as it might seem. How many of their employees actually do get admitted to hospital more quickly as a result of private insurance? Illness is most often experienced by those who have chronic ailments, or those who have retired. Chronic illnesses are not covered by medical insurance and the employer has little interest in providing medical cover for those who have retired. If insurance premiums continue to rise, employers will begin to question what sort of service they are getting from the NHS, particularly in view of the fact that the NHS frequently under-utilizes its surgeons.

Perhaps employers should re-examine their premiums to see if they are indeed 'paying twice' for one service. Perhaps direct negotiations with their local health authorities, to ensure better use of the money that industry pays in taxes, would eventually enable them to save considerable sums on expensive private insurance premiums.

Exposure and public hanging!

One method of changing behaviour amongst a group of people is to isolate one or two who are clearly misbehaving and to make an example of them by some well publicized punishment. The principle here is that this public examination and humiliation of one person's wrongdoing will discourage others from following in a similar vein. This line could be pursued with consultants and managers in order to identify two or three individuals who were clearly in breach of the guidelines on devoting substantially the whole of their time to the NHS. It might have the effect, if the punishment was particularly severe, of making the whole profession re-think its stance towards private practice during the normal working day.

The argument against such a policy is that it unfairly scapegoats one or two individuals who are really, in essence, no different from a substantial group within the set. The result might well be ruined careers for a small number of individuals, and the loss of their operating skills to the NHS. Such action would not, of itself, achieve the overall aim of changing the working practices of all surgeons, but it might then force a greater consideration of the need for a full-scale national enquiry examining the actual workload of surgeons in both the NHS and private sectors. The results of such a study would either show that there was no significant problem in terms of breach of contract or, alternatively, if breaches were found to be widespread, a 'debt repayment' system could be enacted by insisting that those surgeons who had 'short-changed' the NHS undertook extra cases in the NHS to make up for the workload that they have previously failed to undertake.

Re-entry of the churches into hospital care

In a recent book, Terry Waite (1993) referred to work he had undertaken for a medical missionary society of the Roman Catholic Church. The Church had been responsible for establishing some of the major hospitals in towns and cities throughout the Third World, originally for the benefit of the whole community, but particularly for the poor. Over the years these hospitals had become major providers of health care, but increasingly were the centres of private practice and a service which was biased towards the rich. The problems that the Roman Catholic Church encountered throughout the world, 5 or 10 years ago, now confronts churches in England today. Religious order hospitals frequently, although not exclusively, are involved in the provision of care for those who are insured or who can pay privately. The time might now have come for the churches to withdraw entirely from the provision of private health care. There can be no religious ethic that would support the earlier treatment of one patient ahead of another simply on the grounds of ability to pay.

The church could also consider going a step further. Given that the current market situation leads to an increasingly two-tiered service, it might now be time for churches to re-enter the health care market on behalf of the poor. If the existing health care system remains intact, then one assumes that the government would be only too delighted to see new providers coming into the market and the church's emphasis on care and service could establish a formidable opponent to inefficiently run NHS hospitals and 'private for profit' hospital organizations.

TIME FOR CHANGE

My generation of angry young men had a spokesman in the prolific song writer Bob Dylan. I am no longer young, but I remain angry. The question Dylan raised in 1962 still needs asking today: 'How many times can a man turn his head, pretending he just doesn't see?' The inequality faced by one group is easily identified as being caused by the self-interest and even greed of others. We are the others and we need to ask questions of ourselves.

- Managers and politicians need to re-examine the two-tier system which offers a worse service to the poor than to the rich.
- Surgeons need to reconsider whether they will take money from, and give priority to, those who have a lower clinical need than others.

- Patients need to be more assertive in fighting for a more efficient service from the NHS, rather than buying their way out of pain and worry at the expense of others.

The results of achieving change could be breathtaking – faster treatment for the poor, less need for the rich to pay twice and, possibly, less unnecessary surgery, particularly amongst the rich. Such success will only be achieved with considerable difficulty. Higher productivity in the NHS will mean more state expenditure unless there is a reduction in the number of surgeons or, more profitably, a huge drive to reduce unnecessary surgery.

A tale of two cities?

The first city will never provide a comprehensive service, but it pretends it can. The second city wants a comprehensive service, but finds itself frustrated by having to support a parasite which uses its resources to sell the easy parts of health care to the other city. How long will managers, politicians and surgeons continue to allow health care to be allocated according to ability to pay, thus forcing citizens into two cities? How long will it be before the citizens of the second city fight for independence?

Appendix, references and index

CONTENTS

APPENDIX

THE CASE FOR AN ENQUIRY

The evidence presented in this book suggests that there are sufficient grounds to doubt that we are making the best use of our highly' trained surgical manpower. Politicians, surgeons and health service managers are challenged to undertake a systematic review of the workload of consultant surgeons in the NHS and the private sector. Is workload adequate and fairly distributed and, if not, why not?

I suggest that an enquiry be undertaken in two parts. Equity and efficiency are just two of the important criteria of a health care system and sometimes there has to be a trade off between the two. It might, therefore, be wise to start by pursuing each independently before worrying about the link. I suggest that an enquiry into equity should be led by consumer representatives, whilst an enquiry into efficiency be made by surgeons, managers and the Department of Health. The two parts of the enquiry should be conducted within one calendar year and should be published simultaneously. Only when the results are publicly available should decisions be made about the need (if at all) to change the structure of the NHS and the private sector in Britain.

Part 1 – a consumer enquiry

This work should be conducted by representatives of patients' organizations and consumer associations, possibly supported by charitable funds. It should have one observer from the medical profession and one observer from either the Health Service managers or the Department of Health. Ideally, the survey should be comprehensive and cover all surgeons in Britain. A more focused alternative would be to select for study only surgeons whose NHS clinics have a wait of 3 months or more.

Part 2 – a professional enquiry

This study of surgical activity should be undertaken by representatives of the medical profession, managers and the Department of Health, with two outside observers from the consumer enquiry. Ideally, this study would cover all surgeons in Britain, but could commence, as a pilot study, in two regions, or, alternatively, select only those surgeons with out-patient waiting times in excess of 3 months or in-patient waiting lists of over 100 patients. The study could be either prospective, retrospective or both.

TASKS FOR THE CONSUMER ENQUIRY

1. Survey all hospitals and health authorities to obtain data about each surgeon. This should include a schedule of all NHS clinics and private rooms sessions, schedule of all NHS operating lists, a list of all private hospitals where operating is conducted, contractual status in the NHS, out-patient waiting time for an NHS clinic and waiting times for appointment in the private sector.
2. Analyse data collected to determine the extent of:
   - the difference in waiting time between the two sectors
   - the amount of private sector activity that takes place during normal working hours by consultants with full-time and maximum part-time contracts
   - the link between long waiting times and the level of provision of surgeons and clinics in the locality.
3. Display the information for each locality through the local media:
   - to enable local managers, surgeons and patients to verify the accuracy of the data
   - to help GPs and patients 'shop around' for short waiting times.
4. As a further means of verifying the data recruit 'wait watchers' – patients and relatives who will send information to a hotline. They will look out for differences in waiting time experience between the private sector and the NHS and give information about the time of day they were offered or received NHS and private consultation or operative treatment.

5. In the event of non-cooperation from hospitals, consider publishing details of non-compliance and select a small number of areas for detailed investigation.
6. Establish a panel to take written and verbal evidence from any patients, surgeons or managers who wish to comment on the issue.

TASKS FOR THE PROFESSIONAL ENQUIRY

1. Collect basic data for each individual surgeon about:
   - every operation conducted in a 6 month period, whether it be NHS or private (the details of each operation should include status of patients – NHS or private; type of hospital – NHS or independent; date of operation and time of day if recorded; type of operation; BUPA classification; and time taken if recorded)
   - number of new patients seen in consultant NHS clinics
   - number of new patients seen in private rooms
   - contractual commitment of each consultant
   - schedule of all NHS clinics and operating sessions
   - schedule of all private rooms sessions and a list of all hospitals used for private operating.
2. Analyse data to determine:
   - whether or not there is any relationship between NHS and private practice volume (both for in-patients and out-patients)
   - whether or not the volumes of activity undertaken are acceptable professional practice
   - whether or not low volumes are caused by inadequate levels of resources (e.g. too small a number of clinics or theatre sessions made available).
3. Publish the results of the analysis, not naming individual surgeons, but showing the volume of individuals in a coded form, both in terms of the number of operations performed and the number of new out-patients seen. The data should also be displayed in a standardized form to take account of the complexity and time spent on operation.

References

Abel-Smith B 1964 The hospitals 1800-1948: a study in social administration in England and Wales. Heinemann Educational Books Ltd., London: p. 480

Allen P 1993 Medical and dental staffing prospects in the NHS in England and Wales 1992. Health Trends 25(4): 118–126

American Child Health Association 1934 The pathway to correction in physical defects. ACHA, New York: p. 80

Ancram M A F J K 1994 Parliamentary question. Parliamentary Debates (Hansard) House of Commons January 24: 236, 67

Anderson F 1988 IHSM drops queue jump plan after angry reception. Health Service Journal June 2: 605

Anon. 1986 Queue for operations may move to London. Birmingham Post, December 4

Anon. 1993 Deaths after surgery: doubts on value of a 'league table'. Letters to the Editor The Times September 11: 17

Anon. 1994 Health Service Journal 20 October: 4

Anon. 1994 The unhealthy poor The Economist June 4: 27–28

Audit Commission 1994a Protecting the public purse 2: probity in the public sector. Combating fraud and corruption in the NHS. Unpublished draft circulated for consultation

Audit Commission 1994b Protecting the public purse 2: ensuring probity in the NHS. HMSO, London

Audit Commission 1995 The doctors' tale: the work of hospital doctors in England and Wales. HMSO, London.

Beckett M 26 January 1995 Parliamentary question. Parliamentary Debates (Hansard) House of Commons: 243, 342

Beecham L 1994 Royal colleges produce evidence of reduced activity. British Medical Journal March 5: 661

Beecham L 1994 Consultants consider sanctions over local pay. British Medical Journal 309: 1600-1601

Bevan G, Devlin B 1994 All free health care must be effective: limiting medical practice variation. Social Market Foundation Memorandum No. 4

Bottomley V 1987 Parliamentary question Parliamentary Debates (Hansard) House of Commons November 24: 123, 179

Bottomley V 1988 Parliamentary question Parliamentary Debates (Hansard) House of Commons March 9: 129, 244

Brindle D 1994 NHS 'raises £170m from private beds'. The Guardian November 21: 7

British Association of Otolaryngologists 1986 Workload for consultant otorhino-laryngologists. The Royal College of Surgeons of England, London

British Medical Association Orthopaedic Subcommittee of Central Committee for Hospital Medical Services undated Model job description for consultant posts in orthopaedic and traumatic surgery. BMA, London

Brook R H 1994 Appropriateness: the next frontier. Appropriateness ratings could revolutionise health care. British Medical Journal 308: 218–219

Bulstrode C 1995 Embarrassing greed? British Medical Journal 310: 198–199

Bunker J P, Barnes B A, Mosteller F (eds) 1977 Costs risks and benefits of surgery. Oxford University Press Inc., New York

Byrne A J 1991 Private hospitals and waiting lists. Health Service Journal March 14: 8–9

Campling E A, Devlin H B, Hoile R W, Lunn J N 1993 The report of the National Confidential Enquiry into Perioperative Deaths. 1991–92 London The Royal College of Surgeons of England, NCEPOD

Chadda D 1994a Private practices. Health Service Journal February 10: 12–13

Chadda D 1994b Sir Duncan's move to BUPA board is greeted with anger and surprise. Health Service Journal September 29: 7

Churchill W quoted in Democracy in the National Health Service discussion paper prepared for the joint Wales Trade Union Congress-Wales Socialist Medical Association Conference Llandrindod Wells October 30 1976

Clouston E 1994 HIV surgeon may be disciplined. The Guardian December 27: 3

College of Ophthalmologists 1988 Hospital eye service. College of Ophthalmologists, London

Coulter A, Klassen A, MacKenzie I Z, McPherson K 1993 Diagnostic dilation and curettage: is it used appropriately? British Medical Journal 306: 236-239

Davidge M G, Harley M, Vickerstaff L, Yates J 1987 The anatomy of waiting lists. The Lancet 1: 794–796

Davie R, Butler N, Goldstein H 1972 Report of the National Child Development Study (1958 cohort): From birth to seven. The National Children's Bureau, Harlow, Longman

De Melker R A 1993 Treating persistent glue ear in children: more patience less surgery. British Medical Journal 306: 5–6

Dean M 1993 Distinction awards versus market pay. The Lancet 341: 1354

Department of Health 1990 Consultants' contracts and job plans. Health Circular HC(90)16

Department of Health 1991 Government response to the first report from the Health Committee Session 1990–91 Public expenditure on health services: waiting lists. Department of Health, London: Cm1586

Department of Health 1993a Assessing the effects of health technologies principles practice proposals. Report of the Advisory Group on Health Technology Assessment Department of Health, London

Department of Health 1993b Hospital episode statistics England: financial year 1989–90. Government Statistical Service, London

Department of Health 1995 The Patient's Charter and You. Department of Health, London

Department of Health NHS Management Executive 1992 Hospital waiting list in-patients and day cases: England at 31 March 1992. Department of Health Information Division, Stanmore

Department of Health and Social Security 1979a Pay and conditions of service: contracts of consultants and other senior hospital medical and dental staff. Personnel Memorandum PM(79)11 Annex 'A': The whole-time/maximum part-time option

Department of Health and Social Security 1979b Pay and conditions of service: contracts of consultants and other senior hospital medical and dental staff. Personnel Memorandum PM(79)11 Annex 'B': 1975 Letter from Secretary of State for Social Services to Dr Derek Stevenson April 17

Department of Health and Social Security 1979c Pay and conditions of service:

contracts of consultants and other senior hospital medical and dental staff. Personnel Memorandum PM(79)11

Department of Health and Social Security 1986 Handbook on the management of private practice in Health Service hospitals in England and Wales Distributed under cover of Health Circular HC(86)4 Health Services management: private practice in Health Service hospitals 1986 March

Devlin B 1994 Patients' Charter: a surgeon's view. Prime cuts in the body politic. The Guardian December 14 : 6

Donaldson L J 1994 Doctors with problems in an NHS workforce. British Medical Journal 308: 1277–1282

Doyle C 1994 Rationing in action The Daily Telegraph September 13: 18

Dylan B 1962 Blowin' in the wind. Copyright M Witmark & Sons

Editorial 1992 Private grief. Health Service Journal June 4: 16

Editorial 1993 The true story of NHS delays. The Independent September 10

Financial Secretary to the Treasury 1990 Treasury Minute on the Nineteenth to Twenty-fifth and Twenty-seventh Reports from the Committee of Public Accounts 1989–90 HMSO London: Cm 1247

Finkel M L (ed.) 1988 Surgical care in the United States: a policy perspective. The Johns Hopkins University Press, Baltimore

Fletcher D 1994 Private cash boost for trust hospitals. The Daily Telegraph March 16: 4

Frankel S, West R (eds) 1993 Rationing and rationality in the NHS: the persistence of waiting lists. Macmillan, London

George S, Brazier J 1991 Information needs in a provider market: a case-study of ENT. Journal of Public Health Medicine 13(2): 108–114

Ghouri N 1994 A day in the death of the NHS. London Evening Standard January 17: 23

Gillard M 1994 Hospital was doomed say doctors. The Observer December 11: 2

Glover J A 1938 The incidence of tonsillectomy in school children. Proceedings of the Royal Society of Medicine XXXI: 1219–1235

Gray D, Hampton J R, Bernstein S J, Kosevoff J, Brook R H 1990 Audit of coronary angiography and bypass surgery. The Lancet June 2: 1317–1320

Hannan E L et al 1991 Coronary artery bypass surgery: the relationship between in-hospital mortality rates and surgical volume after controlling for clinical risk factors. Medical Care 29: 1094–1107

Havers N, Danziger D 1994 I thought: 'It can't be cancer'. The Independent January 31: 18

Higgins J 1988 The business of medicine: private health care in Britain. Macmillan Education Ltd., Basingstoke

Hoare J 1992 Tidal wave new technology medicine and the NHS. King's Fund Centre, London

Hoffenberg R 1994 Letter to the editor. The Times August 4: 17

House of Commons Committee of Public Accounts 1990 The NHS and independent hospitals. Twenty-eighth Report. HMSO, London

House of Commons 1994 Committee of Public Accounts: Eighth Report Session 1993–94. The Proper Conduct of Public Business. HMSO, London

House of Commons Early Day Motion No. 415 1995 Treatment of private patients by NHS surgeons laid down by Tessa Jowell MP January 18

House of Commons Health Committee 1991 Public expenditure on health services: waiting lists. First Report. HMSO, London

House of Commons Welsh Affairs Committee 1991 Elective surgery Volume I. Sixth Report. HMSO, London

Jones J 1995 Sick pay price as doctors put faith in hunches. The Observer February 5: 8

Laing W 1992a UK private specialists' fees – is the price right? Norwich Union Healthcare Ltd., Norwich

Laing W 1992b Going private: independent health care in London. King's Fund London Initiative, London

Laing's Review of Private Healthcare 1993. Laing & Buisson Publications Ltd., London

Langlands A 1995 A vision beyond winners and losers. Health Service Journal February 2: 10–11

Laurance J 1993 Figures highlight high-risk hospitals. The Times September 8: 1

Laurance J 1995 Doctors say NHS damaged by private practice. The Times January 20: 2

Lee-Potter J 1995 Dying from a bad case of dogma. The Independent January 20: 18

Letter 1991 West Midlands RHA Regional Managing Director to Regional General Managers Ref KFB/CDS/AEP February 27

Lewis B V 1993 Diagnostic dilation and curettage in young women should be replaced by outpatient endometrial biopsy. British Medical Journal 306: 225–226

Lewis E B 1981 Private practice. British Medical Journal 282: 841

London Implementation Group 1993 Report of the Cardiac Specialty Review Group. HMSO, London

Luft H, Bunker J, Enthoven A 1979 Should operations be regionalised? An empirical study of the relation between surgical volume and mortality. New England Journal of Medicine 301: 1364–1369

Luft H S, Garnick D W, Mark D H 1990 Hospital volume physician volume and patient outcomes: assessing the evidence. Health Administration Press, Ann Arbor, Mitchigan

Luke chapter 16, verse 13

Marshall J, Narula A A 1993 Persistent glue ear in children (letter). British Medical Journal 306: 454

Mawson S R, Stroud C E 1972 The indications for tonsillectomy and adenoidectomy. Health Trends 4: 31–32

Monopolies and Mergers Commission 1994a Private medical services: a report on agreements and practices relating to charges for the supply of private medical services by NHS Consultants. HMSO, London; Cm 2452

Monopolies and Mergers Commission 1994b Private medical services: a report on agreements and practices relating to charges for the supply of private medical services by NHS Consultants. HMSO, London; Cm 2452 Appendix 4.7: 237

Mordue A, Parking D W, Baxter C, Fawcett G, Stewart M 1994 Thresholds for treatment in cataract surgery. Journal of Public Health Medicine 16(4): 393–398

National Audit Office 1989 The NHS and independent hospitals: report by the Comptroller and Auditor General. HMSO, London

Nicholl J P, Thomas K J, Williams B T, Knowelden J 1984 Contribution of the private sector to elective surgery in England and Wales 1981. The Lancet July 14: 89–92

Nicholl J P, Beeby N R, Williams B T 1989 Role of the private sector in elective surgery in England and Wales 1986. British Medical Journal 298: 243–247

Office of Population Censuses and Surveys 1990 Tabular list of the classification of surgical operations and procedures. Fourth Revision. HMSO, London

O'Leary D P, Collins C D 1994 Analysis of a year's general surgical activity in a District General Hospital. Annals of The Royal College of Surgeons of England (Suppl.) 76: 176–181

Owen D 1976 In sickness and in health: the politics of medicine. Quartet Books, London

Page M 1993 The Good Doctor Guide. Simon and Schuster, London

Personal communication 1987 December 9

Personal communication 1988a October 20

Personal communication 1988b December 13

Personal communication 1988c December 14

Personal communication 1994a September 20

Personal communication 1994b

Personal communication 1995 February 10

Personal communication undated D K Nicol to Hospital Consultants and Specialists Association

Phillimore P, Beattie A, Townsend P 1994 Widening inequality of health in northern England 1981–91. British Medical Journal 308: 1125–1128

Powell J E 1976 Medicine and politics: 1975 and after. Pitman Medical Publishing Co Ltd., Tunbridge Wells

Pozo J L, Jones C B 1993 What is a reasonable orthopaedic surgical workload? An analysis of elective and trauma workloads using two different complexity scoring systems. Annals of The Royal College of Surgeons of England (Suppl.) 75: 152–157

Primarolo D 1994 US care could damage your health. The Guardian August 18: 20

Rogers L 1994 Doctors claim three in four operations are unnecessary. The Sunday Times November 27: 1

'Shepherd J F 1994 Surgical removal of third molars: prophylactic surgery should be abandoned. British Medical Journal 309: 620–621

Sherman J 1990 Consultants warned on abusing NHS contracts. The Times May 5

Shrimsley R 1994 Waldegrave defends half-truth: when it is acceptable to mislead MPs – by the Minister for Open Government. The Daily Telegraph March 9: 1

The British United Provident Association Ltd. 1993 Working with BUPA: a guide for specialists. Section 1, Schedule of procedures. BUPA, London

The British United Provident Association Ltd. 1994 Clinical care analysis: sharing information with the medical profession. BUPA, London

The Institute of Health Services Management undated Statement of primary values. IHSM, London

The Medical Directory 1993. Longman Group UK Ltd., Harlow

The Royal College of Surgeons of England 1990 General surgical workload and the provider/purchaser contract: notes for guidance. RCSE, London

Timmins N 1994 Ministers in U-turn over 'health gap'. The Independent May 4: 7

Townsend P, Davidson N (eds) 1982 Inequalities in health: The Black Report. Penguin Books Ltd., Harmondsworth

Vallance-Owen A 1994 Backbone of the NHS. Hospital Doctor November 17: 12

Waite T 1993 Taken on trust. Hodder & Stoughton, London

Wilkin D, Dornan C 1990 General practitioner referrals to hospital: a review of research and its implications for policy and practice. Centre for Primary Care Research Department of General Practice University of Manchester, Manchester

Williams B T, Nicholl J P 1994 Patient characteristics and clinical caseload of short stay independent hospitals in England and Wales 1992–3. British Medical Journal 308: 1699–1701

Williams M H, Frankel S J, Nanchahal K, Coast J, Donovan J L 1994a Cataract surgery. In: Stevens A and Raftery J (eds) Health care needs assessment: the epidemiologically based needs assessment reviews. Radcliffe Medical Press, Oxford. Vol 1: pp 658–659

Williams M H, Frankel S J, Nanchahal K, Coast J, Donovan J L 1994b Total hip replacement. In: Stevens A and Raftery J (eds) Health care needs assessment: the epidemiologically based needs assessment reviews. Radcliffe Medical Press, Oxford. Vol 1: p 464

Williams M H, Frankel S J, Nanchahal K, Coast J, Donovan J L 1994c Hernia repair. In: Stevens A and Raftery J (eds) Health care needs assessment: the epidemiologically based needs assessment reviews. Radcliffe Medical Press, Oxford. Vol 2: pp 1–77

Williams M H, Frankel S J, Nanchahal K, Coast J, Donovan J L 1994d Total knee replacement. In: Stevens A and Raftery J (eds) Health care needs assessment: the epidemiologically based needs assessment reviews. Radcliffe Medical Press, Oxford. Vol 1: p 524

Winslow C M, Kosekoff J, Chassin M R et al 1988 The appropriateness of performing coronary artery bypass surgery. Journal of the American Medical Association 260: 505–509

Wood B, Wong Y K, Theodoridis C G 1972 Paediatricians look at children awaiting adenotonsillectomy. The Lancet September 23: 645–647

Yates J 1987 Why are we waiting? Oxford University Press, Oxford

Yates J 1995a Serving two masters: consultants, the National Health Service, and private medicine. A Dispatches Report for Channel 4 Television January 18

Yates J 1995b Serving two masters: consultants, the National Health Service, and private medicine. Channel 4 Television, London, and Inter-Authority Comparisons and Consultancy Health Services Management Centre University of Birmingham

Yates J, Wood K 1985 Out-patient waiting time. Inter-Authority Comparisons and Consultancy, Birmingham

Index